MEDICA...

Passing t...

Second ...ition

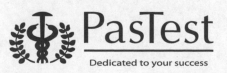

PasTest

Dedicated to your success

MEDICAL FINALS
Passing the Clinical
Second Edition

Christopher E.G. Moore Bsc (Hons) MBBS, PhD, FRCP
Consultant Clinical Neurophysiologist
St Mary's Hospital
Portsmouth

Anna M.T. Richardson BSc (Hons) MB ChB MRCP(UK)
Consultant Neurologist
Greater Manchester Neuroscience Centre
Hope Hospital
Salford

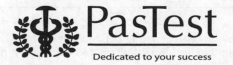

PasTest

Dedicated to your success

© 2005 PASTEST LTD
Egerton Court
Parkgate Estate
Knutsford
Cheshire
WA16 8DX

Telephone: 01565 752000

First Published 1996
Second Edition 2005

Reprinted 2007

ISBN: 19011 98634
ISBN: 978 1901198 638

A catalogue record for this book is available from the British Library.

The information contained within this book was obtained by the author from reliable sources. However, while every effort has been make to ensure its accuracy, no responsibility for loss, damage or injury occasioned to any person acting or refraining from action as a result of information contained herein can be accepted by the publishers or author.

PasTest Revision Books and Intensive Courses
PasTest has been established in the field of postgraduate medical education since 1972, providing revision books and intensive study courses for doctors preparing for their professional examinations. Books and courses are available for the following specialties:

MRCGP, MRCP Parts 1 and 2, MRCPCH Parts 1 and 2, MRCPsych, MRCS, MRCOG Parts 1 and 2, DRCOG, DCH, FRCA, PLAB Parts 1 and 2.

For further details contact:
PasTest, Freepost, Knutsford, Cheshire WA16 7BR
Tel: 01565 752000   Fax: 01565 650264
Email: enquiries@pastest.co.uk   Web site: www.pastest.co.uk

Text prepared by Vision Typesetting Ltd, Manchester
Printed and bound in the UK by MPG Books Limited, Cornwall, UK

CONTENTS

Contents

INTRODUCTION TO THE SECOND EDITION

Since the publication of the first edition of Medical Finals: Passing the Clinical in 1996 medical education in general, and assessment of competence in particular, has undergone a sea change. Although there is at present a heterogeneous approach among medical schools in England, Scotland and Wales, generally speaking the 'old' long case, short case and viva have been replaced by hopefully more objective measures of assessment, such as the objective structured long examination record (OSLER) and objective structured clinical examination (OSCE). Vivas are often reserved for honours and borderline pass/fail students in some universities. The Mini CEx is also gaining popularity.

Therefore, it may seem strange that the content of the cases in this second edition remains largely the same as in the first edition, that the long cases are still represented and have been added to, and that the book has not significantly grown in size – as happens with many second editions. We feel that while the methods of examination have changed, the clinical signs and symptoms have not. A student's ability to demonstrate competence still relies on good communication skills with the patient and examiner, an understanding of a structured clinical examination, and the ability to recognise physical signs and put them into context.

The book has been significantly revised in its organisation, and all cases and viva questions related to one system are now grouped together without the long/short distinction. We hope that this will allow for easier location and revision planning. There is however, an index of long cases for those of you who wish to look at the important long cases in isolation.

We have labelled some of the more obscure cases as hard (rare/advanced/honours) so that valuable time is not wasted by starting with these. We hope that the book will remain popular and act as a concise review of the majority of cases seen in medical examinations, whatever the method of assessment and whatever the stage of medical education.

As always, we hope you find the book useful and wish you luck in the examination and your future careers.

THE PATIENTS

In-patients

Most patients will have stable conditions and will not be very unwell at the time of the examination. You will not see someone on the day they experience a myocardial infarction but you may see them a few days later before discharge, especially if they have a murmur, rub or evidence of heart failure. While 'on the wards' make sure you get a feel for the kind of patients who would be suitable/well enough for transfer to another ward for a morning of examination.

While some patients will have been admitted as an emergency with an acute illness, others may well have been admitted electively, with regards to a specific complication arising in the course of an established disease. Introduce the case accordingly.

Many of your teachers are examiners as well, so find out which kinds of patient they like to examine on, ask them how they assess students and what their favourite viva questions are.

Out-patients

In the weeks before examinations we (consultants and our medical teams) are asked to look out for patients with noteworthy physical signs whom we will see in our clinics and to ask them if they would come in to help with examinations. This is often a prime time to attend extra clinics as part of revision.

Actors as patients

Increasingly in some medical schools, actors are used in final-year examinations to test history-taking skills. There will be an examiner sitting close by. You will be typically given an introductory scenario, such as, 'Mrs Jones has been complaining of headaches for the last two months', and instructed to take a history and ascertain a specific diagnosis. The actor will have been well versed in the clinical features of the particular disorder (eg the headache of raised intracranial pressure secondary to a space-occupying lesion/migraine) and will give you the 'right' answers if you ask the right questions!

This type of station might be viewed as somewhat easier than others. Be prepared for it, and do not allow yourself to feel intimidated. The actor may have been instructed to come across as tense (anxiety neurosis), irritable (hyperthyroid, hypoglycaemic) or tearful (depression), and you will be judged on your ability to handle such a situation, as well as on your diagnostic skills (put the patient at ease, reassure them, etc.). If the actor asks you difficult questions, don't guess. Politely say that you are uncertain, but that you will ask advice from your senior colleagues. You are being examined as to your competence to take up position as a foundation year one junior doctor, not a consultant physician!

HOW TO USE THIS BOOK AND PASS

Buy your own copy! This increases our retirement fund and allows you to scribble all over it.

Use the syllabus checker to find the gaps in your knowledge and confidence.

Think of a patient with long-standing diabetes and a house full of complications: How many cases can you cover? (Answer by email please.)

Go through each system of examination and practise on both your colleagues and your patients.

Seek out patients with relevant conditions and review their signs.

Learn how to become a confident (not arrogant) human being. This will facilitate your interpersonal skills and therefore your technique in the examination.

ACKNOWLEDGEMENTS

FIRST EDITION

We would like to thank the many colleagues who have given us useful tips while producing this book and especially those who have taught us over the years, in particular:

Stephen Brecker, Senior Registrar, Cardiology; Terry Wardle, Consultant Physician; Jon Shaffer, Senior Lecturer, Gastroenterology; George Lipscombe, Senior Registrar, Medicine; Andy Higham, MRC Training Fellow; Matthew Lewis, Registrar, Gastroenterology; Wolfgang Schady, Senior Lecturer, Neurology; Tony Heagerty, Professor of Medicine; Claire Pulford, Lecturer, Geriatric Medicine; Chris Rickards, Senior Registrar, Neurology; David Neary, Professor of Neurology; Eve Russell, Senior Registrar, Psychiatry; Peter Goulding, Consultant Neurologist; Mike Davies, Senior Lecturer in Medicine; Malcolm Littley, Consultant Physician: Mohammed Akil, Senior Registrar, Rheumatology.

Responsibility for the accuracy of this text is of course our own.

We would also like to acknowledge the support of our families: Teddy, Dan, Lucie, Matthew and Keith.

SECOND EDITION

Many people have helped us over the past 7 years in the progression of our careers both as clinicians and as researchers and personally. Of our colleagues not previously mentioned Dr David McKee, consultant neurologist, wrote the HIV case for us. We thank Drs Mark Roberts, Ruth Seabrook, Claire Pulford, Angelica Wiek, David Holder, Peter Heath, Max Lyons-Nandra and Louis Merton. Kath, Julie, Anna, Jo, Gill, Christina, Pauline, Julie and Trudy also deserve mention.

We are pleased with the continued support of PasTest, in particular Lorna Young, Nicky Paris and Kirsten Baxter whose patience has been much appreciated. We would also like to acknowledge the support of friends and family, in no particular order: Keith,

Acknowledgements

Matthew, Joe, Dan, Teddy, Cheryl, Charlotte, James, Lila, Gill, Sarah, Richard, Thomas, Will, Alex, Ben and Matty.

I would like to dedicate my efforts to the memory of my father Michael whom sadly died a few years ago (CM).

ABBREVIATIONS

Most abbreviations used in this book are explained when they first appear. The common abbreviations are listed below.

ACTH	adrenocorticotropic hormone
AIDS	Acquired Immune Deficiency Syndrome
ALT	alanine transaminase
AMA	anti-mitochondrial antibody
ANA	anti-nuclear antibody
AST	aspartate transaminase
BP	blood pressure
CABG	coronary artery bypass graft
CEx	Clinical Examination
CNS	Central Nervous System
CT	computed tomography
CVA	cerebrovascular accident
CVS	cardiovascular system
CXR	chest X-ray
dsDNA	double-stranded DNA
DVT	deep vein thrombosis
ECG	electrocardiogram
ESR	erythrocyte sedimentation rate
FBC	full blood count
HIV	Human Immunodeficiency Virus
HOCM	hypertrophic obstructive cardiomyopathy
iv	intravenous
JVP	jugular venous pressure
LFT	liver function test
MCS	microscopy, culture, sensitivity
MCV	mean cell volume
NSAID	non-steroidal anti-inflammatory drug
OCP/HRT	oral contraceptive pill/hormone replacement therapy
PE	pulmonary embolism
RA	rheumatoid arthritis
RhF	rheumatoid factor
sc	subcutaneous
SIADH	syndrome of inappropriate ADH
SLE	systemic lupus erythematosus
SMA	smooth muscle antibody

Abbreviations

SOB	shortness of breath
SVCO	superior vena caval obstruction
TB	tuberculosis
TFT	thyroid function test
TIA	transient ischaemic attack
U&E	urea and electrolytes
USS	ultrasound scan
VF	vocal fremetis
WCC	white cell count

Normal values

Albumin	35–55 g/l
Alkaline phosphatase	30–130 IU/l
Aspartate aminotransferase	5–27 IU/l
Bicarbonate	24–30 mmol/l
Bilirubin	2–13 μmol/l
Calcium	2.15–2.65 mmol/l
Chloride	93–108 mmol/l
Creatinine kinase	0–170 IU/l
Creatinine	55–125 μmol/l
Erythrocyte sedimentation rate	0–10 mm (first hour)
γ-Glutamyl transferase	0–30 IU/l
Haemoglobin (men)	13.5–17.5 g/dl
Haemoglobin (women)	11.5–15.5 g/dl
Mean corpuscular volume	76–98 fl
Phosphate	0.80–1.4 mmol/l
Platelet count	$150–400 \times 10^9$/l
Potassium	3.8–5 mmol/l
Sodium	136–149 mmol/l
Thyroid-stimulating hormone	0.8–3.6 mU/l
Thyroxine	70–160 nmol/l
Total protein	65–80 g/l
Urea	2.5–6.5 mmol/l
Vitamin .B$_{12}$	200–900 pg/ml
White blood count	$4–11 \times 10^9$/l

Syllabus checker

As an aid to revision you can use this syllabus as your own personal checklist. You should aim to achieve at least two ticks per case before the date of the examination. *Hard cases.

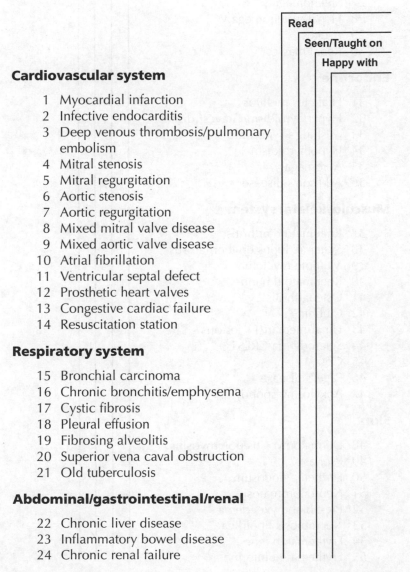

Read

Seen/Taught on

Happy with

Cardiovascular system

1 Myocardial infarction
2 Infective endocarditis
3 Deep venous thrombosis/pulmonary embolism
4 Mitral stenosis
5 Mitral regurgitation
6 Aortic stenosis
7 Aortic regurgitation
8 Mixed mitral valve disease
9 Mixed aortic valve disease
10 Atrial fibrillation
11 Ventricular septal defect
12 Prosthetic heart valves
13 Congestive cardiac failure
14 Resuscitation station

Respiratory system

15 Bronchial carcinoma
16 Chronic bronchitis/emphysema
17 Cystic fibrosis
18 Pleural effusion
19 Fibrosing alveolitis
20 Superior vena caval obstruction
21 Old tuberculosis

Abdominal/gastrointestinal/renal

22 Chronic liver disease
23 Inflammatory bowel disease
24 Chronic renal failure

	Read	Seen/Taught on	Happy with

25 Nephrotic syndrome
26 Hepatomegaly
27 Splenomegaly
28 Hepatosplenomegaly
29 Ascites
30 Renal masses

Endocrine

31 Diabetes mellitus
32 Hyperthyroidism/Graves' disease
33 Cushing's syndrome
34 Hypothyroidism
35 Acromegaly
36 Addison's disease

Musculoskeletal system

37 Rheumatoid arthritis
38 Systemic lupus erythematosus
39 Multiple myeloma
40 Rheumatoid hands
41 Osteoarthritis
42 Clubbing
43 Ulnar/median/T1 lesions
44* Scleroderma/CREST
45 Gout
46 Paget's disease
47 Ankylosing spondylitis

Skin

48 Dermatomyositis/polymyositis
49 Psoriasis
50 Erythema nodosum
51 Neurofibromatosis
52* Pre-tibial myxoedema
53 Necrobiosis lipoidica
54 Erythema ab igne
55* Erythema multiforme

	Read	Seen/Taught on	Happy with

56 Vitiligo/pityriasis
57* Hereditary haemorrhagic
telangiectasia

Neck

58 Goitre
59 Lymphadenopathy
60 Jugular venous pressure

Neurology

61 Stroke
62 Multiple sclerosis
63* Motor neurone disease
64 Parkinson's disease
65* Myotonic dystrophy
66* Myasthenia gravis
67 Syringomyelia
68 Spastic paraparesis
69 Peripheral neuropathy
70 Myopathy
71 Absent ankle jerks and extensor
plantars
72 Pes cavus
73 Cerebellar syndrome
74 Gait abnormalities

Visual fields

75 Homonymous hemianopia
76 Bitemporal hemianopia
77* Central scotoma
78* Tunnel vision concentric
constriction

Pupils

79* Horner's syndrome
80* Holmes–Adie pupil
81* Argyll Robertson pupil

Read

Seen/Taught on

Happy with

Eye movements

82 Nystagmus
83* Ataxic nystagmus
84 IIIrd nerve lesion
85 Ptosis
86 VIth nerve lesion
87 Thyroid eye disease
88* Congenital squint

Fundi

89 Diabetic fundus
90 Hypertension
91 Optic atrophy
92 Papilloedema
93 Retinal pigment

Other cranial nerves

94 VIIth nerve palsy
95* Cavernous sinus syndrome
96* Cerebello-pontine angle lesion
97* Jugular foramen syndrome
98 Bulbar palsy
99 Pseudobulbar palsy
100* The 3 Ds

Psychiatry

101 Depression
102 Psychosis/schizophrenia
103 Anorexia nervosa
104 Substance abuse

HIV/AIDS

105 HIV infection/AIDS

THE LONG CASE

INTRODUCTION TO THE LONG CASE

Candidates are usually given 45–60 minutes to take a history from and examine a patient. This is followed by 15 minutes for presentation and discussion. Do not be surprised if you are taken back to the patient to demonstrate the physical signs you have elicited.

Do ensure that you allow yourself at least five minutes at the end to prepare yourself and your notes before going in to see the examiners. Write a summary of the salient features in the history and the examination, and your differential diagnosis. It is wise to prepare in advance a list of the investigations you would perform together with appropriate treatment as these are the questions most likely to be asked by the examiners.

It is important to establish a good rapport with the patient. Introduce yourself, explain how important the examination is to you, what you have to do and how much time you have. Try to make the patient feel that they are on your side against the examiner – this way they will try to help you as much as possible early on. Find out if the patient is an in-patient or an out-patient. If he or she is an in-patient find out when they were admitted and why. Often patients in the examination have chronic conditions and are under routine follow-up: in these cases the presenting complaint may go back many years and it is best to go over the history chronologically and then concentrate on the major current problems. Don't forget to ask the patient if they know their diagnosis!

Remember that you are expected to perform a full physical examination, including measurement of blood pressure and possibly urinalysis. Occasionally the patient in the long case will have no abnormal physical signs.

The examiners might expect you to present the case fully – be clear and concise, avoiding long lists of negative findings. Volunteer a short summary at the end rather than waiting to be asked. Be prepared, however, for the examiner instead to plough straight in with questions regarding your differential diagnosis and management plan. A good start may be one such as this, 'I have been to see Mrs Smith, a 53-year-old lady, who is currently an in-patient at this hospital under the care of Professor Jones'. Then either, 'She was well until two weeks ago when she presented with acute central chest pain ...' or 'She has a 15-year history of rheumatoid arthritis and was admitted last week for investigation of anaemia ...'.

Be courteous at all times – to patients and examiners alike.

LONG CASE INDEX

Listed below are popular long cases that appear frequently in examinations. Those in bold are covered in detail in this book as they are the most common/important.

Cardiovascular system

Chest

Abdominal/gastrointestinal/renal

Musculoskeletal/haematology

THE LONG CASE

Presenting complaint (PC)
History of the presenting complaint (HPC)
Past medical history (PMH)
Family history (FH)
Drug history (DH)
Review of systems (ROS)
Social history (SH)
Clinical examination
Summary

PC   Remember to use the patient's words – not your interpretation of them. Patients rarely complain of melaena/haemoptysis/dysarthria, etc.

HPC   For each symptom you need to ascertain the following:
Onset – sudden or gradual duration.
Pattern – continuous or episodic. If episodic the frequency and duration of individual episodes.
Course of illness to date – Static / Progressive / Improving.
Precipitating / Aggravating / Relieving factors.
Associated symptoms.
Once you have questioned the patient fully regarding the PC, specifically ask the other questions relating to that particular organ system, eg if patient complains of shortness of breath and cough, ask specifically about Sputum / Haemoptysis / Fever / Chest pain.

PMH   This is straightforward.
Ask specifically about past Medical / Surgical / Psychiatric histories.
Ask specifically about Hypertension / Diabetes / Asthma / Tuberculosis/ Rheumatic fever.

FH   Record details of all first-degree relatives (Parents / Siblings / Children).
Record the age at death / Cause of death / Related illnesses.

DH   Use proprietary names rather than brand names.
                Record the Dose / Dose frequency / Duration of
                prescribed medication.
                Record recent changes in medication, especially those
                made during this inpatient stay.
                Ask specifically about allergies and their nature.

ROS   Briefly ask questions pertaining to each organ system.
                Always ask about Weight loss / Appetite / Fever / Rash /
                General well-being.

SH   Smoking habit – smoker/ex-smoker/life-long non-
                smoker.
                Alcohol consumption – see Case 104 for more details.
                Occupation and previous occupations/unemployment.
                Marital status – Married / Single / Divorced / Widowed /
                Dependants.
                Wage / Income support / Invalidity benefit / Other
                allowances.
                House / Bungalow / Flat / Steps, and Driving ability.
                Activities of daily living – Washing, Dressing, Eating /
                Eliminating, Shopping, Socialising, Home Help /
                District Nurse.

Examination
For the long case you will be expected to perform a **full** physical
examination, including **blood pressure measurement** and
sometimes **urinalysis**. Although examination techniques for all the
relevant systems are included in this book, you need to devise your
own routine and be comfortable with it, avoiding unnecessary
repetition and ensuring nothing is missed out. For example:

General appearance   Well / Unwell / Febrile
                                        Distressed / Dyspnoeic / In pain
                                        Pale / Jaundiced
                                        Cachectic / Obese

Hands
Face
Neck
Chest (CVS/resp)

Abdomen
Nervous system
Musculoskeletal system
Urinalysis

THE SHORT CASE

INTRODUCTION TO THE SHORT CASE

You will see a number of patients and will be given various instructions. Two examiners will take you around, usually for about 30 minutes, in which time you may see four to six cases. The types of case will usually be balanced between the systems; it would be unusual for a candidate not to be asked to examine the cardiovascular system. OSCE examinations follow a similar pattern.

You will be assessed on:
your approach to the patient
your ability to perform a careful competent examination
your ability to pick up important signs
your ability to interpret these signs.

Your approach to the examiners is not formally tested but if good can only help in their overall assessment of you.
It is VERY important that you are polite to the patients, ask their permission to examine them and do not hurt them.

APPROACH TO THE PATIENT

A good start may sound like this:
Examiner: 'Please examine this man's heart.'
Candidate to the patient (making good eye contact with the patient and shaking their hand): 'How do you do sir? I am Mr Smith. Would you mind if I examined your heart? '
Patient: 'No.'
Candidate: 'Please would you take off your top and lean back on the pillows ... Are you comfortable? ' Observe face etc. 'May I feel your pulse? '

APPROACH TO THE EXAMINERS

On first meeting the examiners make sure you introduce yourself. Try to answer the question asked and not something else. During your short cases you may be encouraged to keep up a running commentary. If you have never done this before, practise it now. You may be allowed to continue uninterrupted but more often than not you will be stopped and started. This can be frustrating, but if you are prepared for it you should not allow it to disrupt your examination routine.

When you have finished examining the patient, thank them, make sure they are covered and then turn fully to face the examiners, try not to look away from them. Good eye contact and body posture help to present a competent appearance. Look at the spot at the top of the examiner's nose and let rip! 'On examining Mr Smith's cardiovascular system, I have found evidence of mitral regurgitation without mitral stenosis that is not complicated by heart failure or infective endocarditis. This is evidenced by ....'

If you are not so sure about the diagnosis try: 'I am uncertain about the definitive diagnosis but my differential diagnosis is that of an ejection systolic murmur. Aortic stenosis is unlikely as the pulse character is normal, mitral regurgitation may be present but there is no radiation to the axilla. The other possibility is aortic sclerosis which is common in a man of this age.'

Each short case included in this book gives the main clinical features that may be present and some of the associated findings. We feel the cases included are the commonest conditions seen in exams. We will have missed some cases that you or your teachers think relevant, however, if you are familiar with all these cases you should have little trouble in picking up most of the important features during the examination.

The 'Teaching points' and 'Comments' give some associated and hopefully relevant facts. Many of these facts will be needed to answer extra questions during the clinical and also to answer those asked during the viva-voce.

THE SPOT DIAGNOSIS

Don't be surprised if, instead of being asked to go through the examination of a system, you are simply asked to look at a patient, or perhaps ask him or her some questions and then come up with the diagnosis. Don't panic.

Certain conditions lend themselves to spot diagnosis and tend to come up again and again. Often these are either endocrine or neurological conditions. Most of these conditions should be familiar to you; if not, make sure you recognise them from picture atlases or find patients with them on the wards or in the clinics.

Cases on spot diagnosis:

THE VIVA

The viva can be a very frightening experience as the whole of the medical syllabus is up for discussion. This is usually made worse by your supposed friends who often do their best to 'psych' you out in the days and minutes leading up to the event.

A few tips are listed below that can make things easier during the examination. There are several ways of gaining valuable experience during your clinical training.

- Arrange to have a mock viva.
- Act as a helper if your hospital runs a MRCP course.
- Ask the consultants who teach you about their favourite viva questions.
- Ask previous candidates about their experiences BUT get them to remember the common topics as well as the rarities.

During the viva:
- Use good body language (good eye contact/hands held on or below table).
- Speak clearly/do not mumble.
- Answer the question asked.
- If you do not understand the question say so at once.
- If you know nothing about the subject under discussion say so at once – either you will be given a clue or the subject will be changed.
- If in doubt about something return to first principles (if you can remember them).
- Make sure you know about the management of emergency situations (cardiac arrest/acute asthma/anaphylaxis/hypovolaemic shock etc.).

When given the situation of an ill person follow this protocol:

Examiner: 'You are called to casualty to see a patient who is comatose ...'

Candidate: 'I would go immediately to the patient and perform resuscitation as needed, paying attention to Airway, Breathing and Circulation and I would assess their consciousness level using the Glasgow Coma Scale.'

This is usually enough for the examiner to set up the case in more detail, 'OK. He is breathing spontaneously and has a BP of 110/175, heart rate 85, what would you do next?'

Candidate: 'I would check his blood glucose and look for small pupils, a sign of opiate overdose.'

When asked how you would manage a patient, follow this protocol:

Examiner: 'How would you manage a patient with .... syndrome?'
Candidate: 'First of all I would confirm the diagnosis by taking a full history, performing a complete physical examination and arranging appropriate investigations.' This shows you are thorough in your approach to a patient. Then if you know a specific treatment go on with, 'Specific treatment for this condition would be with ... .' If you don't know the specifics you could try, 'Treatment in general can fall into conservative/medical/surgical/palliative. In this case medical drug therapy would be the first option ... .'

When asked the causes of a particular condition, go through your medical sieve.

VITAMIN D:
V	Vascular
I	Infective (bacterial/viral/fungal/protozoal/other)
T	Traumatic
A	Auto-immune/connective tissue
M	Metabolic/endocrine
I	Iatrogenic
N	Neoplastic (benign/malignant/primary/secondary)
D	Neuropsychiatric Degenerative/ageing

When asked about a particular condition, follow a slightly different plan:

Dressed	Definition
In	Incidence/prevalence
A	Age
Surgeon's	Sex
Gown	Geography
Anaesthetists	Aetiology
Perform	Pathology; Macroscopic/microscopic (Light/electron)
Deep	Diagnosis made on **History**
	Examination
	Investigation
Coma	Clinical features Complications (see below)
To	Treatment (conservative/medical/surgical/palliative)
Perfection	Prognosis

When asked about complications, think through each body system in turn:

CVA / RS / GIT / GUT / CNS / Haematological / Immune / Musculoskeletal

As in any examination a degree of luck always helps. We hope your quota arrives for the day – good luck.

The cases

The cases

CARDIOVASCULAR SYSTEM

CARDIOVASCULAR SYSTEM
'Examine this patient's heart'

Introduce and expose
> Patient comfortable, reclining at 45 degrees

Observe   Pallor
Dyspnoea / Cyanosis

Hands   Clubbing (42)
Splinter haemorrhages   Endocarditis
Peripheral cyanosis   Cool peripheries
Tendon xanthomata   Hyperlipidaemia
Tar staining

Pulse (radial)
> Rate
> Rhythm
> Radio-femoral delay in young adults (coarctation of the aorta)
> Check specifically for collapsing pulse (7)

Blood pressure
> Tell the examiner 'At this stage I will usually measure the blood pressure'. If you are lucky you will be told what it is.

Neck   Carotid pulse   Volume / Character / Thrill
JVP   Height   ↑ + pulsatile in right heart failure
↑ + non-pulsatile in SVCO (20)
Waveform   Giant systolic V waves in tricuspid regurgitation (7)
May displace ear lobes

Face   Anaemia
Xanthelasma
Corneal arcus
Malar flush

With patient sitting back

Praecordium

Inspect   Scars   Median sternotomy (coronary artery bypass graft (CABG) / Valve replacement)
Lateral thoracotomy (mitral valvotomy)

Apex visible

Palpate   Localise apex beat
Tapping   Palpable valve closure
Heaving   Sustained contraction
Thrusting Hyperdynamic contraction
Thrills and parasternal heave

Percuss

Not usually performed

Auscultate
1. At apex with bell
2. Turn patient onto left hand side
   Relocate apex and listen specifically for mitral stenosis (4) (held expiration)
   Turn patient back
3. At apex with diaphragm
   If murmur listen for radiation into axilla
4. Listen in all other areas
   Left sternal edge
   Pulmonary
   Aortic
5. Listen to carotids (If no aortic murmur, ? isolated carotid bruit)

Sit patient forward

Praecordium

Listen specifically for the early diastolic murmur of aortic regurgitation (7) at left sternal edge in held expiration.

Lungs   Listen at lung bases for inspiratory crackles.

Sacrum   Feel for sacral oedema while asking the patient 'Does this hurt? This should alert the examiner to the fact you have looked for sacral oedema.

Feel for ankle oedema

Tell the examiner 'To finish my examination I would like to see the temperature chart and dip the urine' (? endocarditis).

When presenting your findings comment on the valve lesion(s) and whether it is complicated by heart failure or endocarditis, eg 'This lady has mitral stenosis, as evidenced by the mid-diastolic murmur heard loudest at the apex in held expiration, which is complicated by atrial fibrillation but not heart failure or endocarditis.'

Comment
Left-sided murmurs increase in held expiration, right-sided with inspiration.

Case 1:
MYOCARDIAL INFARCTION

Appears fairly frequently as a long case; it is a common condition and patients are usually relatively well and able to give a clear story.

PC	**Chest pain** (usually)	
	Sometimes no chest pain but SOB	
	Collapse / Sweating	

HPC	Pain	**Central** / Radiation to neck / Jaw / Teeth / Arms (one or both, usually LEFT)
		Crushing / Squeezing / Tight / 'Like a band'
		Occasionally felt as radiation only (no pain at all in the chest)

Typically at rest / May be brought on by Unusual Exercise / Argument / Intercourse / Snow shovelling, etc.
Pain is prolonged / Often relieved only by opiate analgesia
Associated symptoms include SOB / Sweating / Nausea / Vomiting / Pallor / Greyness
Ask about any chest pain or SOB since admission

PMH Ask about previous vascular disease
                Angina – present in about 40%
                Claudication
                Cerebrovascular disease (61)
Hypertension / High cholesterol / Diabetes

FH Particularly a history of ischaemic heart disease in first-degree relative.

DH Prior to and since admission.
Was the patient put on a drip (thrombolysis)? Are they now on aspirin?

ROS Chest pain / SOB / Swelling of calves

SH **Smoking habit** – before admission.
Employment may be profoundly affected, eg HGV drivers banned from driving if follow-up exercise test reveals abnormal findings after full thickness infarct.

EXAMINATION
General appearance
> Anaemia / Xanthomata / Xanthelasma / Corneal arcus / Tar staining / Pyrexia

CVS Atrial fibrillation (10) (Common post-myocardial infarction (MI))
Bradycardia (heart block / β-blocker treatment)
Blood pressure (BP) often low post-MI
Presence of fourth heart sound is very common
Look for signs of left ventricular failure (13)
Poor cardiac output / Basal crackles / Dyspnoea
Evidence of peripheral vascular disease
Absent pulses / Femoral bruits / Carotid bruits

INVESTIGATIONS
> Troponin T levels
> FBC
> ESR
> (Both WCC and ESR may be elevated)
> U&E / Glucose
> Cholesterol
> ECG
> CXR

TREATMENT
Remember BOOMAR
> **B** Bed rest
> **O** Oxygen
> **O** Opiate analgesia
> **M** Monitor for arrhythmias
> **A** Anti-coagulate (subcutaneous heparin to prevent deep vein thrombosis (DVT))
> **R** Reduce the size of the infarct with thrombolytic drugs

Stop smoking

COMPLICATIONS

Early   Cardiac arrhythmias
Cardiac failure
Pericarditis
Recurrent infarction / Angina
Thrombo-embolism
Mitral regurgitation (chordae rupture)
Ventricular septal / Free wall rupture

Late   Cardiac failure (13)

Dressler's syndrome	Weeks to months post-MI / Auto-immune pericarditis / Fever / Pericardial effusion Treatment non-steroidal anti-inflammatory drugs (NSAIDs) / Steroids / Not anti-coagulants

Ventricular aneurysm

Comment:
Advice to give patient on discharge

Stop smoking
Review diet especially if overweight
Exercise   Daily short walks (×2) 15–20 minutes duration
        Increase distance gradually
Avoid strenuous exercise
Avoid driving for 6 weeks
Sexual intercourse best avoided for 1 month
Most patients should aim to return to work 3 months later
Some occupations that may be affected:
        HGV / Public service vehicle driving
        Airline pilot

All patients will be on aspirin (or alternative antiplatelet agent), nearly all on a cholesterol lowering agent, and the most will will be on a beta-blocker + / – ACE inhibitor.

Case 2:
INFECTIVE ENDOCARDITIS

An uncommon condition, but patients are usually in hospital for several weeks, and therefore appear relatively frequently in exams.

PC   Fever
         Constitutional symptoms
         Symptoms of cardiac failure (13) / Embolisation

HPC   Characteristically in infective endocarditis, at least in the sub-acute form, the symptoms are of such gradual onset that the patient often finds it impossible to date the onset of their illness.
         Predisposing factors include previous dental and surgical procedures, so remember to ask specifically. The mean interval between the procedure and the diagnosis being made is 3 months.
         Together with the fever there may be symptoms of sweats, chills or, rarely, rigors.
         Symptoms of general malaise, anorexia, weight loss, aching joints etc. are often prominent – note their rather non-specific nature.
         Occasionally the condition may present with complications secondary to embolisation, eg stroke.

PMH   Around 50% are known to have pre-existing valve disease.
         Ask for history of rheumatic fever / St Vitus' Dance (chorea)

EXAMINATION
General appearance
         Fever / Pallor / Evidence of weight loss
         Petechial haemorrhages – Trunk / Limbs / Mucous membranes
         Splinters / Haemorrhages
         Osler's nodes
         Janeway lesions (looks like blotchy palmar erythema)
         Roth spots (retinal haemorrhages with pale centre)
         State of teeth / ? Dentures

CVS   Tachycardia / heart failure

Murmur – Most commonly aortic regurgitation or mitral regurgitation

Abdomen
Splenomegaly

Urinalysis
Microscopic haematuria and proteinuria

INVESTIGATIONS
Blood cultures ×6
Echocardiography to look for
Vegetations / Valve damage
FBC – Mild normochromic, normocytic anaemia (chronic disease picture)
ESR – Elevated
U&E

TREATMENT
Treatment of any underlying infection, eg dental abscess
Intravenous bactericidal anti-biotics, according to results of blood cultures
Surgery for extensive valvular damage / Prosthetic valve infection / Severe heart failure (13)

COMPLICATIONS
Embolisation (from the vegetations)
Stroke (61)
Renal infarction
Splenic infarction (splenic rub)
Osler's nodes
Immune complex formation
Glomerulonephritis (proteinuria)
Roth spots (retina)
Janeway lesions

Comment:
Prosthetic valves

Endocarditis on prosthetic valves (12) accounts for up to one-third of all cases. Early infection – within 2 months of surgery – carries a particularly high mortality. Established infection will cause alteration of the prosthetic valve sounds – 'muffling' them.

Intravenous drug users are at risk of developing **right-sided** endocarditis; usually the tricuspid valve is affected. Typically the patient is a young man, with no known history of heart disease and a fairly short history. In these cases embolisation commonly causes pulmonary infarction ± abscess formation.

Case 3:
DEEP VENOUS THROMBOSIS / PULMONARY EMBOLISM

DVT/PE are common conditions, and can be the primary illness leading to hospital admission or, more commonly, arise as a complication during hospital admission, eg post-MI.

PC   Calf pain / Swelling.

HPC   Gradual progression over a few days.
Ask about preceding risk factors, eg air travel, fractures, any cause of relative immobility.
Is the patient pregnant?
Ask specifically about SOB, chest pain, haemoptysis.

PMH   Previous DVT?
History of of 'white leg' in pregnancy?

FH   Very important.
Certain clotting deficiencies are familial.

ROS   Is the patient taking oral contraceptive pill (OCP) / hormone replacement therapy (HRT).
Since admission, has patient been on daily sc injections (heparin), tablets given at tea-time (warfarin).

SH   Smoking habit (predisposes to hypercoagulable state).

EXAMINATION
General appearance
    Dyspnoeic / Bruising (iatrogenic)

Legs   Calf asymmetry (measure)
    Tenderness
    Erythema
    Oedema
CVS   Sinus tachycardia (often the only sign of a PE)

Respiratory
> Tachypnoeic   Oxygen treatment
> Pleural rub

INVESTIGATIONS
> Clotting profile (prothrombin time (PT) / Activated partial thromboplastin time (APTT)) before treatment
> If recurrent, seemingly unprovoked or positive family history perform detailed thrombophilia screen.
> Doppler ultrasound scan of calf.
> D-Dimers
> If PE suspected needs spiral CT or ventilation / Perfusion (V/Q) scan

TREATMENT
> TED stockings
> Mobilise
> Anticoagulation (see viva answer)

Comment
Most patients will be discharged on warfarin, to be taken for several months. It is very important to advise patients to inform all concerned medical practitioners, dentists, chemists, etc. that they are taking warfarin. Warfarin has many drug interactions. Patients should be asked to seek immediate medical advice if they develop spontaneous bleeding or widespread bruising. All patients should be given a warfarin information card prior to discharge and avoid cranberry juice!

Case 4:
MITRAL STENOSIS

Introduce and expose

Observe	? Female
Hands	
Pulse	**Atrial fibrillation (10)**
BP	Low with normal pulse pressure
Neck	JVP may be increased
	Giant V waves
Face	**Malar flush** (cyanosis and telangiectasia)
Praecordium	
Inspect	? Left thoracotomy scar (mitral valvotomy)
Palpate	Undisplaced tapping apex beat?
	Parasternal heave
Auscultate	**Loud first heart sound**
	Opening snap
	With bell, low-pitched rumbling **mid-diastolic murmur** at apex
	? Murmur of tricuspid regurgitation
Lung bases	Usually clear
Ankle oedema	Yes, if right heart failure present

TEACHING POINTS
Causes
Essentially only one – rheumatic fever
NB Rheumatic mitral stenosis is much commoner in women.

Comment
If asked for details of treatment mention digoxin for associated atrial fibrillation, anti-coagulants for prevention of systemic embolisation from left atrial thrombi and diuretics for any associated right heart failure, as well as mitral valvotomy and mitral valve replacement.

Case 5:
MITRAL REGURGITATION

Introduce and expose
Observe
Hands   Splinters
Pulse   Sinus rhythm or atrial fibrillation
BP
Neck
Face
Praecordium
  Inspect   Visible apex beat
  Palpate   Displaced / **Thrusting** apex beat / Systolic thrill
               Parasternal heave (due to large left atrium)
  Auscultate   Soft first heart sound / **Third heart sound** /
               Pansystolic murmur at apex / Radiation to axilla
Lung bases
Ankle oedema

TEACHING POINTS
Causes

1. **Ischaemic heart disease**	Secondary to left ventricular dilatation (functional) Papillary muscle ischaemia / Infarction
2. **Rheumatic heart disease**	(Previous mitral valvotomy for mitral stenosis)

3. Mitral valve prolapse
4. Infective endocarditis

There are many others, eg the connective tissue diseases (SLE, RA), ankylosing spondylitis, Marfan's, hypertrophic obstructive cardiomyopathy (HOCM).

Comment
It is sometimes difficult to give a definitive diagnosis when listening to an ejection systolic / pansystolic murmur so be sure to work out the features of the four main differential murmurs: aortic stenosis (AS) / Mitral regurgitation (MR) / Aortic sclerosis / ventricular septal disease (VSD).

Case 6:
AORTIC STENOSIS

Introduce and expose
Observe   Male
Hands
Pulse   Sinus rhythm
BP   Low systolic with **narrow pulse pressure**,
                 eg 110 / 90 mmHg
Neck   Carotid pulse
                 Low-volume / Slow-rising / Thrill
Face
Praecordium
  Inspect   Visible apex beat
  Palpate   Undisplaced **heaving** apex beat
                 Thrill over aortic area
  Auscultate   Harsh **ejection systolic murmur** loudest in aortic
                 area
                 Often heard easily at apex / Radiates to **carotids**
                 Soft second heart sound (may be absent)
Lung bases   Normal if uncomplicated case

Pedal oedema

TEACHING POINTS
Symptoms   1. Chest pain
                 2. Shortness of breath
                 3. Syncope

Causes   1. Bicuspid valve and degeneration
                 2. Rheumatic
                 3. Congenital (young patient)

Investigations ECG (Left ventricular hypertrophy) / CXR
                    Echocardiogram
                    Cardiac catheterisation

Comment
In elderly people calcification of a normal valve can produce a
murmur which is similar, but the pulse, BP and apex will be normal
– so called **aortic sclerosis**.

Bicuspid valve occurs in 1% of the population, and is commoner in
males. With increasing age the valve becomes increasingly fibrotic
and calcified, and hence aortic stenosis most commonly presents
in men aged 40–60 years.

Case 7:
AORTIC REGURGITATION

Introduce and expose

Observe	Check for features of Marfan's* / Ankylosing
spondylitis	
Hands	Splinters / Rheumatoid hands / Arachnodactyly
Pulse	Sinus rhythm / **Collapsing**
BP	**Wide pulse pressure**, eg 180 / 60 mmHg
Neck	Large volume carotid pulse / Easily seen in neck (not JVP)
Face	High-arched palate / Argyll Robertson pupils (81)

Praecordium

Inspect	Visible apex beat
Palpate	Displaced / **Thrusting** apex beat
Auscultate	Soft / blowing
	Early diastolic murmur at the left sternal edge
	Loudest sitting forward in held expiration
	NB There is always, in addition, a systolic murmur due to the increased flow across the aortic valve. There may be a mid-to-late diastolic murmur (Austin Flint) due to the back flow onto the mitral valve.
Lung bases	Normal in the uncomplicated case
Ankle oedema	

*High-arched palate / Span > height / Arachnodactyly / Risk of aortic dissection

TEACHING POINTS

Causes	1. Rheumatic fever
	2. Infective endocarditis
	3. Ankylosing spondylitis
	4. Rheumatoid arthritis
	5. Marfan's syndrome*
	6. Syphilis

Comment
There are a number of eponymous signs characteristic of, although rarely seen, in aortic regurgitation. They are beloved of examiners:
De Musset's sign: the head nods with each pulsation
Quincke's sign: capillary pulsation visible in the nail beds
Corrigan's sign: vigorous arterial pulsations seen in the neck.

Case 8:
MIXED MITRAL VALVE DISEASE

It is quite common, at least in exams, to see patients with mixed mitral valve disease, ie with signs of both mitral stenosis and mitral regurgitation.

Remember that, as for lone mitral stenosis, rheumatic heart disease is essentially the only cause.

Two reasons for mixed mitral valve disease:
1.   Excessive valvular damage
2.   Previous mitral valvotomy – **look for the lateral thoracotomy scar**.

If you are doing particularly well (or you are particularly unlucky), you may be asked to comment on the predominant valve lesion.

	Predominant mitral stenosis	**Predominant mitral regurgitation**
Apex	Tapping	Displaced/ thrusting
First heart sound	Loud	Soft
Third heart sound	Absent	Present
Atrial fibrillation	Common	

Comment
Remember: the third heart sound represents rapid ventricular filling, and therefore is obviously incompatible with significant mitral stenosis.

Case 9:
MIXED AORTIC VALVE DISEASE

Essentially two causes:

1. Rheumatic heart disease
2. Infective endocarditis on a previously stenotic valve

Remember: even in lone aortic regurgitation you should expect to hear a systolic murmur due to increased flow across the valve. However, there will not be any signs of aortic stenosis.

	Predominant aortic stenosis	Predominant aortic regurgitation
Pulse	Slow-rising	Collapsing
Apex	Heaving	Displaced/thrusting
BP Systolic pressure	Low	High
Pulse pressure	Narrow	Wide

Comment
A bisferiens pulse is characteristic of mixed aortic valve disease.

Case 10:
ATRIAL FIBRILLATION

Although atrial fibrillation may be isolated be careful of associated mitral stenosis and hyperthyroidism.
If it is atrial fibrillation (AF) alone, you will likely to be asked to just feel the pulse and you may well be asked for causes.

Introduce and expose
Observe	? Obviously hyperthyroid
Hands	Sweating / Tremor
Pulse	**Irregularly irregular** in rhythm and in volume (? Rate over one full minute)
BP	
Neck	Goitre
Face	Malar flush
Praecordium	
Inspect	
Palpate	
Auscultate	Again count rate over a full minute Note varying intensity of first heart sound
Lung bases	
Ankle oedema	

TEACHING POINTS
Causes
1. Ischaemic heart disease
2. Mitral valve disease
3. Hyperthyroidism
4. Pneumonia
5. Cardiomyopathy
6. Constrictive pericarditis
7. 'Lone'
+ many others

Comment
The presence of a pulse–apex deficit means that the atrial fibrillation is **uncontrolled**.
Digoxin – the usual treatment does not alter the underlying rhythm, but simply controls the ventricular rate.
Patients with non-rheumatic AF should be anti-coagulated to decrease the risk of future stroke.

Case 11:
VENTRICULAR SEPTAL DEFECT

This is the commonest congenital heart lesion; the patient is often young.

Introduce and expose
Observe   Young, generally well
Hands   Splinters (rare)
Pulse
BP
Neck
Face
Praecordium
  Inspect
  Palpate   Apex undisplaced / Systolic thrill at left sternal
                 edge
  Auscultation   Loud **'tearing' pansystolic murmur** at left sternal
                 edge / Heard well at apex
Lung bases
Ankle oedema

TEACHING POINTS
1. Small ventricular septal defects (VSDs) (**maladie de Roger**) in the absence of symptoms and complications require no treatment.
2. With larger VSDs expect the apex to be displaced, with signs of **pulmonary hypertension** (right ventricular heave / loud P2 / occasionally the extra-diastolic murmur (EDM) of pulmonary regurgitation). These cases will require cardiac catheterisation and surgical treatment.
3. A very large VSD can lead to **Eisenmenger's syndrome** (severe pulmonary hypertension with reversal of the shunt to R > L most often in a young patient). The massively increased blood flow irreversibly damages the pulmonary vessels. The patient will be cyanosed and display finger clubbing. The signs will be those of severe pulmonary hypertension, and the pansystolic murmur (PSM) tends to disappear as the right and left ventricular pressures equalise.

Case 12:
PROSTHETIC HEART VALVES

Prosthetic valves produce a loud closing click and a quieter opening click. A flow murmur across a prosthetic valve is to be expected.

Introduce and expose

Observe	Dyspnoea
Hands	Splinter haemorrhages
Pulse	Atrial fibrillation (mitral valve replacement)
	Collapsing pulse – aortic valve leaking
BP	Wide pulse pressure – aortic valve leaking
Face	
Neck	
Praecordium	
Inspect	Midline thoracotomy scar (both aortic and mitral)
Palpate	
Auscultate	Mitral valve – loud click at first heart sound, opening click in diastole ± mid-diastolic flow murmur
	PSM and signs of heart failure imply valve leakage.
	Aortic valve – Normal first heart sound, ejection click, an ejection systolic flow murmur and loud click at second heart sound
	A collapsing pulse, wide pulse pressure and early diastolic murmur imply valve leakage
Lung bases	
Ankle oedema	

TEACHING POINTS
Complications
> Endocarditis
> Emboli
> Leakage / Congestive cardiac failure (CCF)
> Mechanical dysfunction
> Haemolysis
> Bleeding due to anti-coagulants

Comment

Confusion may be caused if both valves have been replaced. An aortic valve may have been replaced by a pig graft; this does not give rise to abnormal sounds. Always comment on whether the valve is functioning normally (a flow murmur is allowed) or whether it is complicated by leakage / CCF / endocarditis.

Case 13:
CONGESTIVE CARDIAC FAILURE

Cardiac failure can be **left heart failure** where the predominant features are due to poor cardiac output and back pressure on the lungs and **right heart failure** where the features are due to back pressure on the peripheral venous system. The combination of these, ie **biventricular failure**, is termed **CCF**.

Introduce and expose

Observe	**Dyspnoea** / Oedema
Hands	Cool / Peripheral cyanosis
Pulse	Tachycardia / Poor volume
BP	Low
Neck	JVP raised (60), may be behind ear
Face	
Praecordium	
Palpate	Displaced apex beat
Auscultate	Third ± fourth heart sounds
	'Functional murmurs' of mitral and / or tricuspid regurgitation
Lung bases	Inspiratory crackles / Pleural effusion
	Sacral oedema
Ankle oedema	Yes – may extend as far as trunk / Chest wall

TEACHING POINTS

Causes	Ischaemic heart disease
	Valvular heart disease
	Cardiomyopathy (dilated / Restrictive / HOCM)
	Arrhythmias

Comment
High output cardiac failure refers to conditions in which the heart fatigues after excessive pumping of blood, as in arteriovenous shunts or anaemia. It is very uncommon and is almost best forgotten.

Case 14:
RESUSCITATION STATION

Some final year medical examinations, especially those with OSCE-type finals, might include a 'Resus Annie' station. If you have not had the opportunity to practise your resuscitation technique on a dummy, do it now. All hospitals have designated resuscitation officers who love to instruct new recruits.

Your theoretical and practical knowledge will be tested on this station.
You may be asked to proceed as you would if you witnessed a cardiac arrest out of hospital.

Check that the patient is unresponsive.
Check for carotid pulsation.
Call for help.

Then, as in all medical emergencies, think **A B C**.

A   Open the **A**irway, by extending the neck and bringing the chin forward.
B   Give 2 effective **B**reaths.
C   Give 15 external **C**ardiac compressions.

Check for signs of circulation. Continue the cycle (2 breaths, 15 cardiac compressions) until help arrives.

You may also be tested on your knowledge of in-hospital cardiac arrest (after all, if the exam goes well, you will be dealing with them a few months later). Although the above principles still apply, the call for help will be to put out a 'crash call', the airway will be maintained with an endotracheal tube, and breathing with oxygen via an Ambu bag. There should be a team of people, so oxygenation and cardiac compression can be continued simultaneously.

The patient will be attached to a defibrillator monitor, and direct current (DC) shocks administered if appropriate (ventricular fibrillation (VF), ventricular tachycardia (VT)).

All patients are given iv adrenaline (preferably via a central line) while cardiopulmonary resuscitation (CPR) continues. Reversible causes, eg tension pneumothorax, metabolic disturbances, should be sought and corrected.

Don't forget, one member of the team should be trying to ascertain background information (was the patient previously well, any history of cardiac disease, in a young patient any possibility of drug overdose) as well as keeping relatives informed of the situation.

VIVA QUESTIONS
What advice would you give to a patient on discharge having suffered a myocardial infarction?

The areas for advice in this situation can usefully be divided into:

Risk factor identification and management
Lifestyle measures
Pharmacological treatment
Cardiac rehabilitation.

All patients should be strongly advised to stop smoking, eat a healthy diet and exercise regularly. Exercise should be graded, and walking distance and speed gradually increased in the first few weeks.

Almost all patients will have been given an anti-platelet agent (aspirin), a β-blocker and a statin, and many an angiotensin-converting enzyme (ACE) inhibitor. All these agents have been proved to be effective in the secondary prevention of myocardial infarction. The importance of compliance with medication should be stressed to patients.

Programmes of cardiac rehabilitation are of proven efficacy and should be offered to all patients prior to discharge.

Advise patients not to drive for 4 weeks post-MI.

How would you treat deep vein thrombosis?

See Case 3

The main reason for treating deep venous thrombosis is to prevent pulmonary embolism.

Most commonly, low molecular weight heparin (LMWH) is used, which has the advantage of not requiring monitoring. For patients at high risk of bleeding, however 'standard' heparin is more suitable, as its effects can be rapidly terminated by stopping the infusion.

Oral anti-coagulation, with warfarin, should be started at the same time as LMWH – Warfarin takes at least 48–72 hours for its anti-coagulant effect to develop fully. When the international normalised ratio (INR) has been in the therapeutic range (2–3) for 2 consecutive days, heparin can be stopped, and warfarin continued, usually for a period of 3–6 months.

All patients should be given an anti-coagulant card, informing them of the risks and what to look out for (spontaneous excessive bruising, bleeding) and how to seek help.

Warfarin has many drug interactions and it is important that patients are aware that they have to inform all concerned medical practitioners, dentists, etc. of their prescription.

When would you anti-coagulate a patient in atrial fibrillation?

AF is a common arrhythmia, particularly in the over-65 age group. Patients with AF are a high risk group for cardioembolism (from thrombus in the left atrium); patients with AF have a five-fold increased risk of ischaemic stroke. Anticoagulation, with warfarin, has been shown in a number of controlled trials to reduce this risk significantly.

All patients with persistent or paroxysmal AF should be considered for treatment with anti-coagulation, particularly those with a previous history of transient ischaemic attacks (TIAs), stroke or systemic embolism, hypertension or left ventricular dysfunction.

Patient with 'lone' AF probably do not require anti-coagulation, as the risk of cardioembolism is lower in this group.

Obviously, the main drawback of warfarin is the risk of haemorrhage (eg alcohol, falls) and patients at high risk of haemorrhage, eg in alcohol abuse, previous gastrointestinal bleed, falls, should not be treated.

All patients with AF and mitral stenosis need treatment with anti-coagulation, as the risk of cardioembolism is very high in this group.

What is the treatment of congestive cardiac (chronic heart) failure?

Treatment for heart failure aims to improve symptoms and prognosis. Remember, heart failure has a worse prognosis than most cancers.

Obviously treatment in individual cases will depend on the underlying aetiology and severity of the condition.

It is important to exclude other contributory medical conditions, such as anaemia and thyrotoxicosis.

General advice should be given to all patients, regarding stopping smoking, reducing alcohol intake and possibly reducing salt and fluid intake.

The first line of pharmacological treatment is with a diuretic, usually a loop diuretic, such as frusemide. ACE inhibitors are used in most patients. Increasingly selective β-blockers are used in the treatment of heart failure, with care. Arrhythmias should be treated and warfarin given if atrial fibrillation is present. Don't forget to look for valvular disease which might be causing the heart failure, especially aortic stenosis – valve replacement is the treatment. Cardiac transplantation may rarely be necessary.

Tell me about antibiotic prophylaxis in endocarditis.

Patients with valvular lesions, septal defects (atrial or ventricular), prosthetic valves or a previous history of endocarditis, all require prophylactic antibiotics prior to operative procedures or dental treatment (includes scaling as well as extractions).

Oral amoxicillin (3 g) is used most commonly (clindamycin for penicillin-allergic patients). Intravenous anti-biotics are used for patients under general anaesthesia.

The most important step is to inform all patients in the above group to inform all doctors / dentists of their diagnosis, and preferably to carry written information. The precise details of the recommended antibiotic regimens are available in the British National Formulary (BNF).

RESPIRATORY SYSTEM

RESPIRATORY SYSTEM
'Examine this patient's chest'

When asked to examine the chest there are only a few possible diagnoses and you should be able to differentiate between them fairly easily. However, many candidates look ill prepared when it comes to the exam. It is very important to have a strict, well-practised routine (as in all short cases). The examination has six main parts:

Introduce and expose
Ask the patient to remove shirt / blouse (preserve modesty) and sit up at 45 degrees

Observe	Dyspnoea / Respiratory rate	
	Ask the patient to take two deep breaths	
	Watch from halfway down the bed for:	
	1. Asymmetry of chest movement	
	2. Stridor	
	3. Cachexia	
	4. Accessory muscle use / Pursed lips	
Hands	Clubbing (42)	Tumour / Pus (bronchiectasis, abscess) / Fibrosing alveolitis (19)
	Asterixis	Hypercapnia
	Tremor	β-Agonist especially nebulised
	Tar staining	Smoker
	Steroidal skin	Steroid use in Chronic bronchitis / Fibrosing alveolitis / Asthma
	Pulse	Hyperdynamic / Tachycardia
	Hypertrophic pulmonary osteoarthropathy	
	(HPOA) (15)	Tender on squeezing wrist (usually clubbed)
Face	Central cyanosis	Look at tongue
	Cushingoid (33)	
	Horner's syndrome (79)	Apical lung tumour
Neck	Trachea	Pulled to side of collapse / Pushed away from mass / fluid
	JVP	Raised and pulsatile – cor pulmonale
		Raised and fixed – SVCO (20)
	Lymphadenopathy	

Chest   You have to decide whether to examine the front
or the back first. We would suggest the back as
usually all of the possible signs will be there; if so,
you may be told to omit the front thus saving
valuable time and not boring the examiner.

Expansion	Make sure your thumbs are not touching the chest
Percussion	Top to bottom including axillae
Tactile vocal fremitus (TVF)	Use the ulnar border of both hands
Auscultation	Start at apex
Vocal resonance (VR)	

TVF and VR give the same information. VR is more reliable. You
may wish to omit TVF to save time but you should be able to
justify your actions.

Ankle oedema
Extras   Oxygen
Nebulisers / Inhalers

Sputum pot	Purulent = infection / Abscess / bronchiectasis
	Blood = tumour / Infection
Temperature chart	

Comment
At the end of the examination you should be in a position to make a
differential diagnosis of the lung pathology. Try also to note whether
there is right heart failure (cor pulmonale), eg 'This lady is
breathless at rest and has signs of lower zone fibrosis consistent
with a diagnosis of fibrosing alveolitis. There is no evidence of right
heart failure' or 'The raised JVP and ankle oedema suggest this has
been complicated by pulmonary hypertension'.

Case 15:
BRONCHIAL CARCINOMA

PC   Chest symptoms   Worsening cough / Haemoptysis / Chest pain / Hoarse voice / Stridor / Breathlessness / Pneumonia

HPC   Other symptoms   Back pain / Bony pain / Headache (metastatic) / Thirst / Polyuria / Leg weakness / Sensory disturbance / Lethargy

PMH   History of: chronic bronchitis (in view of their common aetiologies) / TB / Pulmonary fibrosis (association with adenocarcinoma)

FH

ROS   Ask about complications of the disease and its treatment.

SH   **Smoking habit** / Passive smoking
Occupation: asbestos / Chromium / nickel exposure

EXAMINATION
General appearance
Cachectic / Breathless / Muscle wasting

Hands   Tar staining / Clubbing

Neck   Lymphadenopathy (59)

Face   Horner's (79) / Hoarse voice (recurrent laryngeal nerve palsy) / SVCO (20)

Respiratory
Pleural effusion (31) / Lobar collapse / Consolidation / May be normal
Radiotherapy marks / Operation scars

Abdomen
　　Hepatomegaly / Ascites
CNS　Papilloedema / Myopathy / Neuropathy / Cerebellar
　　syndrome

Other　There are many non-metastatic complications of
　　malignancy especially with small (oat) cell carcinoma of
　　the lung. You should be familiar with the commonest ones.
　　Cachexia / Weight loss
　　Hypercalcaemia / Hyponatraemia (SIADH) / Ectopic
　　ACTH
　　HPOA
　　Clubbing
　　Polyneuropathy / Autonomic neuropathy / Polymyositis
　　Dermatomyositis / Lambert–Eaton myasthenic syndrome /
　　Cerebellar syndrome
　　Dementia / Myelopathy
　　Thrombophlebitis migrans / Anaemia / Polycythaemia
　　Acanthosis nigricans

INVESTIGATIONS
　　FBC
　　LFTs / Calcium / Sodium
　　CXR
　　Sputum cytology
　　Bronchoscopy / Pleural aspiration / Pleural biopsy
　　Pulmonary function tests (if contemplating surgery)
　　CT thorax
　　(USS abdomen / bone scan / CT brain)

TREATMENT
Surgery Suitable in 20%
　　　　　Attention to　　　Age
　　　　　　　　　　　　Lung function / Hilar and mediastinal
　　　　　　　　　　　　nodes
　　　　　　　　　　　　Metastatic disease / Cell type

Radiotherapy
> Best for squamous cell carcinoma
> Used in those with 'operable' tumour not resected for other reasons
> Palliation for pain / Recurrent haemoptysis / Severe dyspnoea

Chemotherapy
> Reserved for small cell carcinoma

Comment
Three main histological types of bronchial tumour

Squamous
Slow-growing / Metastasises late
Associated with clubbing / HPOA / Hypercalcaemia (due to parathyroid hormone-related protein (PTHrP) release)

Small cell
Fast-growing / Metastases usually present at the time of diagnosis
Associated with SIADH / ectopic ACTH etc.

Adenocarcinoma
Proportionally more common in non-smokers

Case 16:
CHRONIC BRONCHITIS AND EMPHYSEMA

PC   Cough / Sputum / SOB / Wheeze

HPC   History extending back over many years of cough
           productive of scanty mucoid sputum, especially in
           mornings (regarded by many smokers as normal),
           accompanied by increasing SOB and decreasing exercise
           tolerance.
           Admission often precipitated by 'infective exacerbation':
           sputum turns green, increases in amount / SOB / fever, etc.
           Ask specifically about ankle swelling.
           Smoking habit – Smoker / Ex-smoker / Life long non-
           smoker (unlikely)

FH   If the patient is young (< 40 years) may be α_1-anti-trypsin
           deficiency.

ROS   Inhaled / Nebulised bronchodilators (salbutamol /
           Terbutaline)
           Steroids
           Home oxygen

SH   Exercise tolerance when well. Are they able to leave the
           house, shop, etc.?

EXAMINATION
General appearance
           Dyspnoeic / Cyanosed / Febrile / Tar-stained fingers /
           Plethoric

CVS   Cor pulmonale: raised JVP / Loud P2 / Ankle oedema. (The
           parasternal heave is usually obliterated by hyperinflated
           lungs.)

Respiratory

Tachypnoeic

Accessory muscles of respiration / Lip-pursing / Tracheal tug / Recession

Decreased expansion / Increased resonance of percussion note

Quiet breath sounds / Prolonged expiratory phase / Widespread wheezes

Abdomen

Liver often 'pushed down' by hyperinflated lungs.

INVESTIGATIONS

FBC (polycythaemia secondary to chronic hypoxaemia)

CXR

Sputum microscopy / Culture / Sensitivity (MCS)

Pulmonary function tests (peak expiratory flow rate (PEFR) / Forced expiratory volume in 1 second (FEV_1) / Forced vital capacity (FVC))

Arterial blood gases

ECG (looking for changes of right heart 'strain')

TREATMENT

Stop smoking

Bronchodilators

Steroids (only if a significant element of reversibility)

Antibiotics

Controlled oxygen therapy*

Physiotherapy for retained secretions

*It has been shown that long-term oxygen therapy (minimum 15 hours / day at 2 l / min) can reduce mortality in certain patients (those with FEV_1 <1.5 l / Pao_2 < 7.3 kPa / Peripheral oedema).

Comment

Definitions: Chronic bronchitis is a clinical definition – the production of sputum on most days for 3 months of the year in 2 consecutive years.

Emphysema is a pathological diagnosis – enlargement of air spaces distal to the terminal bronchiole, accompanied by destruction of their walls.

It used to be popular practice to divide patients clinically into **blue bloaters** (cyanosed and oedematous with stocky necks) and **pink puffers** (thin and breathless, but not cyanosed). The former were thought principally to have chronic bronchitis and the latter to have emphysema. However this clinical impression has not been borne out by pathological studies, and in fact has more to do with differences in the sensitivity of the respiratory centre.

Case 17:
CYSTIC FIBROSIS

PC	Presenting symptoms	Meconium ileus / Recurrent chest infections
HPC	Method of diagnosis	Sweat test / Lung function / Gastrointestinal absorption
	Chest	Breathless / Sputum / Haemoptysis / Wheeze / Infection Pneumothorax
	GI	Weight loss / Constipation / Cirrhosis (jaundice)
	Cardiac failure	Secondary to pulmonary hypertension / Heart-lung transplant
	Diabetes 10%	
	General	Lethargy in hot weather due to salt loss
	Nasal polyps	
	Decreased fertility	95% azoospermia

Who helps with postural drainage?
How many admissions to hospital?

PMH

Drugs

FH	Autosomal recessive	Gene frequency 1:50 explains 60–70% positive

ROS   Go over any complications not mentioned during the PC.

SH   Problems with schooling / Employment

EXAMINATION
General appearance
Short stature / decreased muscle bulk with severe disease
Clubbing

Chest   Cough (look at sputum) / Pneumothorax / Crackles / Wheeze

CVS   Cor pulmonale: Raised JVP / Ankle oedema / Right ventricular heave

GI   Cirrhosis

INVESTIGATIONS
Sputum culture (Haemophilus / Pseudomonas)
Pulmonary function tests

CXR	Increased lung markings / Consolidation / Pneumothorax
FBC	Anaemia / Increased WCC with infection
U&E	Salt loss / LFTs (? picture of cirrhosis)

TREATMENT
Physiotherapy / Postural drainage
Drugs Pancreatic enzyme supplements / Inhalers / Vitamins
Heart-lung transplant
Gene replacement (experimental at this stage but a very important concept)

Comment
Life expectancy has gradually increased and the mean is now about 35 years.

Case 18:
PLEURAL EFFUSION

This is a common short case and should be well performed.
Introduce and expose

Observe	Chest movement less on affected side / **Cachexia** / Radiotherapy marks
	Mastectomy / Aspiration scars (under the plaster)
Hands	**Clubbing (42)** / Tar stains / Rheumatoid
Face	Cyanosis / SLE butterfly rash
Neck	Lymphadenopathy / Trachea (away from large effusion but towards if co-existing lung collapse)
Chest	Decreased TVF / **Stony dull percussion**
	Decreased breath sounds / Decreased VF
	May have bronchial breathing at upper limit of effusion
Extras	TB (Asian) / Temp chart / Sputum (blood stained) / Ankles (oedema / CCF / DVT / PE)

TEACHING POINTS

Causes	Exudate (protein >30 g/l)	Transudate (protein <30 g/l)
	Tumour (primary/secondary)	Cardiac failure (13)
	PE/infarction	Nephrotic syndrome (25)
	Pneumonia	Cirrhosis (22)
	TB	
	SLE/rheumatoid	
	Diaphragmatic irritation (abscess/pancreatitis)	

Comment

There are many rarer causes. Mesothelioma is usually associated with clubbing and occurs more often after asbestos exposure.
Investigations would include:
CXR / Sputum cytology / Sputum MCS
Pleural fluid analysis / Pleural biopsy
Treatment would include symptomatic drainage and treatment of the underlying condition.

Case 19:
FIBROSING ALVEOLITIS

Introduce and expose

Observe	Dyspnoea / Accessory muscle use / Tachypnoea
Hands	**Clubbing** (60%)
Face	Central cyanosis (if advanced)
Neck	
Chest	Breath sounds – **fine inspiratory crackles**
	Bases > apex
Extras	Oxygen / Cushingoid / Steroidal skin
	Ask to see FEV_1 and FVC measurements

TEACHING POINTS
Other causes of lung fibrosis

Widespread	Upper	Lower
Drugs – Busulfan	TB (21)	Sarcoidosis
Amiodarone	Radiation (Ca breast)	Asbestosis
		Chronic pulmonary oedema
Carcinomatosis	Ankylosing spondylitis	Mitral valve disease (8)
Extrinsic – allergic alveolitis		Silicosis Rheumatoid/ SLE (37, 38)

Comment

FEV_1 and FVC are both reduced causing a restrictive pulmonary deficit. In the absence of an underlying diagnosis, cryptogenic fibrosing alveolitis is the name given. However, there are many auto-immune disorders that are complicated by a similar pulmonary disorder: rheumatoid, SLE, systemic sclerosis, Sjögren's syndrome, polymyositis and chronic active hepatitis. Look out for signs of these.

Case 20:
SUPERIOR VENA CAVAL OBSTRUCTION

Introduce and expose

Observe	Stridor / Dyspnoea
Hands	Clubbed / Tar stained
Face	**Oedematous** / Cyanosed / Puffy eyes
Neck	**Fixed engorged veins** / Lymphadenopathy (59)
Chest	Tortuous veins / Signs of tumour
Extras	Horner's syndrome (79) / Radiation marks

TEACHING POINTS

Causes	**Carcinoma of bronchus**
	Lymphoma
	Mediastinal goitre / Fibrosis

Comment

Urgent treatment with radiotherapy or stenting is required. The patient may complain of **Headaches / Lightheadedness / Syncope**.

Case 21:
OLD TUBERCULOSIS

Introduce and expose

Observe	Patient
	Elderly / Asian / Irish
	Abnormal-shaped chest
Hands	
Face	
Neck	**Trachea to side of collapse**
Chest	Decreased expansion / Old thoracotomy scar / Rib missing
	TVF may be decreased
	Percussion Dull
	Breath sounds Crackles (bronchial breathing)
	VF Decreased

TEACHING POINTS

The signs are variable but are due to **fibrosis and scarring**, leaving areas without working lung tissue. The apex of the lung is most often affected but the signs of apical disease can be difficult to pick up. Beware!

Complications	Fungal mycetoma in cavities
	Malignant change in old scar tissue

Comment

Prior to anti-TB drugs pneumothorax, plombage (ping pong balls put into the chest cavity) and phrenic nerve crush were all used in the treatment of TB. Signs of these may be visible.

VIVA QUESTIONS
When would you instigate long-term oxygen therapy in a patient with chronic bronchitis / emphysema?

The rationale for administering long-term oxygen therapy is to reduce the likelihood of developing pulmonary hypertension and secondary right heart failure (cor pulmonale).

Patients with a PaO_2 < 7.3 kPa when stable are candidates (accept slightly higher PaO_2 if patient has peripheral oedema or signs of pulmonary hypertension). Check PaO_2 in patients with severe airflow limitation (FEV_1 < 30% predicted), those who appear cyanosed, those who have elevated JVP, peripheral oedema and polycythaemia.

Patients should breathe supplemental oxygen for at least 15 hours a day.

Obviously patients should be instructed not to smoke.

What are the risk factors for bronchial carcinoma?

Smoking is the overwhelming risk factor for bronchial carcinoma. Stopping smoking even after many years reduces the risk, and all patients should be strongly encouraged to stop smoking.

Passive smoking is also an important risk factor and future legislation is likely to restrict smoking in public places as an important public health measure.

Exposure to asbestos is fortunately less frequent than previously, but is an important risk factor for mesothelioma.

Tell me about the treatment of TB

TB needs to be treated with combination therapy of several months duration.

It is treated in two phases: an initial phase using at least three drugs and a continuation phase using two drugs. Standard treatment is with rifampicin, isoniazid and pyrazinamide for 2 months followed by 4 months of rifampicin and isoniazid. Drugs for TB are potentially hepatotoxic and liver function should be monitored.

Poor compliance is a particular problem with TB therapy and some patients require supervision when taking their medication, which is then given three times a week.

Treatment is more complex with resistant organisms, in patients with human immunodeficiency virus (HIV) infection and atypical mycobacteria, and requires specialist advice.

Tell me the difference between a transudate and an exudate in a pleural effusion

Pleural effusion means collection of fluid within the pleural space. Pleural effusions can be divided into transudates, protein concentration < 30 g/l, and exudates, protein concentration > 30 g/l. Transudates are secondary to underlying disease, such as heart failure, or medical disorders leading to hypoalbuminaemia (cirrhosis, nephrotic syndrome). Usually there is evidence of the primary diagnosis. Exudates are caused by infection, malignancy, connective tissue disease and pulmonary embolism.

ABDOMINAL, GASTROINTESTINAL AND RENAL

ABDOMEN
'Examine this patient's abdomen'

The key to a successful examination of the abdomen is to look for any extra-abdominal signs to indicate whether there is a problem with liver function, haematological function or both and then go on to find any abdominal signs. By the end of the examination you should be able to tie the two together.

Introduce and expose

Observe	Jaundice	Liver failure
	Wasting	Malabsorption / Malignancy
	Purpura	Hypersplenism
	Pigmentation	Haemochromatosis / Multiple transfusions
	Tattoos	Risk of hepatitis
	Polycythaemia	Polycystic kidneys
	Hyperventilation	Acidosis (renal failure)
Hands	Clubbing	Inflammatory bowel disease
	Leuconychia	Low serum albumin
	Spider naevi	Liver dysfunction
	Asterixis / Tremor	Liver dysfunction
	Palmar erythema	Liver dysfunction
	Dupuytren's	Alcohol / Phenytoin etc.
	Bruising	Clotting function impaired
	Arteriovenous fistula for dialysis (forearm)	
Face	Cushingoid (steroids)	Chronic active hepatitis Transplant Inflammatory bowel disease
	Kayser–Fleischer rings	Wilson's disease
	Jaundice	
	Xanthelasma	Primary biliary cirrhosis Chronic biliary obstruction
	Steroidal	
	Mouth ulcers	
	Parotid enlargement	Alcoholism
Neck	Lymphadenopathy	(Virchow's node)
	Neck feeding line	Malabsorption
	Dialysis line	Polycystic kidneys

Chest   Spider naevi
          Gynaecomastia   (decreased breakdown of
                                oestrogens)
          Sit forward and look for Scars / Sacral oedema / More
          spider naevi
Now ask the patient to lie as flat as possible / Comfortable, one
pillow. Get down to the patient's level.

Abdomen   Do not hurt the patient
          Ask permission / Ask if tender
Inspect   Masses / Ascites / Scars / Striae / Visible peristalsis
          Dilated veins
Palpate   Ask if there is any tenderness before touching
          Masses   Liver / Spleen / Kidneys (see below)
          Inguinal nodes / Hernias
Percuss   Delineate size of masses
          Shifting dullness (ascites) / No need to turn patient if
          not dull
Auscultate Bowel sounds
          Are there any bruits over
          Liver / Mass / Renal artery / Aortic aneurysm
Tell the examiner 'To complete my examination I would usually
examine the external genitalia and perform a rectal examination'.

Legs   Ankle oedema   Low protein states
          Bruising
          Erythema nodosum   Crohn's / Ulcerative colitis
                                  (23)
          Neuropathy   Alcohol / B_{12} deficiency (do
                                  not routinely examine for this
                                  but if there is muscle wasting
                                  suggest that you would)
Extras   Asterixis   Encephalopathy
          Urine   Bile / Protein / blood
          Temperature chart   Infection
          Scratch marks   Cholestasis

Case 22:
CHRONIC LIVER DISEASE

PC Often non-specific: Lethargy / Anorexia / Nausea /Vague abdominal discomfort / Ankle swelling / Easy bruising / Pruritus / Jaundice

HPC Likely to have been non-specifically unwell for some time
Precipitating factors: Haematemesis / Infection / Operations
Previous admissions

PMH Previous episodes of jaundice
Blood transfusions / Intravenous drug use
Auto-immune diseases (32) (associated with chronic active hepatitis (CAH))
Emphysema (α1-anti-trypsin deficiency)
Thrombotic tendency (Budd–Chiari)

FH Enquire carefully
It is crucial to identify treatable causes of chronic liver disease (CLD), eg Haemochromatosis / Wilson's disease

DH May be the cause, eg Methyldopa / Nitrofurantoin (rare)
phenothiazines cause cholestatic jaundice

ROS Amenorrhoea / Impotence / Loss of libido

SH TAKE A CAREFUL ALCOHOL HISTORY (104)
Remember high-risk occupations: Licensing trade / Travelling salesmen / Doctors
Hepatitis risk / IV drug use / Sexuality

EXAMINATION
Most physical findings in CLD are given under the heading 'Examine this patient's abdomen'. It is important to look carefully for any factors that will lead you to the underlying cause of the liver failure, eg Hepatitis / Haemochromatosis / Wilson's disease / Alcohol excess / Tattoos.
The abdominal signs will usually involve **hepatomegaly (26) /**

splenomegaly (27) / ascites (29) (in long-standing cirrhosis the liver is small and shrunken but there will be evidence of portal hypertension). Abdominal scars may reflect Portal shunting / Variceal repair / Transplantation.

Indicators of decompensation

Encephalopathy (decreased detoxification)
Oedema (low albumin)
Ascites
Fetor
Flap / Tremor
Bruising (especially at needle sites)

INVESTIGATIONS

FBC   High MCV
            Low platelets (hypersplenism)
Prothrombin time
LFTs / Albumin
U&E
Hepatitis screen (B and C)
Autoantibodies (anti-nuclear (ANA) / Anti-smooth muscle (SMA) / Anti-mitochondrial (AMA) – primary biliary cirrhosis (PBC))
Immunoglobulins (IgA – alcohol / IgM – PBC / IgG – chronic active hepatitis (CAH))
Iron studies (haemochromatosis)
Abdominal ultrasound / gastroscopy (? varices)
Liver biopsy
α-fetoprotein (hepatocellular carcinoma)
α_1-Antitrypsin level
Copper studies (Wilson's disease)

Comment

Chronic liver disease is the diagnosis you can make at the bedside; cirrhosis is a histological diagnosis, and is made on the results of a liver biopsy. Clotting problems are due to hypersplenism (low platelets) and the lack of liver produced clotting factors (II, VII, IX, X). Factor VII has the shortest half-life hence the prothrombin time is the first to become abnormal.

'Liver function' may be assessed in terms of synthetic function (albumin / Clotting factors) and detoxification (encephalopathy). 'LFTs' enable you to assess hepatocellular damage (high enzyme levels of aspartate aminotransferase (AST) / Alanine aminotransferase (ALT)) or biliary obstruction (raised bilirubin / Alkaline phosphatase).

Case 23:
INFLAMMATORY BOWEL DISEASE

PC   Crohn's disease   Diarrhoea / Abdominal pain /
                                       Weight loss / Malaise
         Ulcerative colitis   Diarrhoea with blood and mucus
                                         / Abdominal pain

HPC   Both diseases are relapsing / remitting in nature, and many
patients enjoy good health most of the time. The patient in
the exam, however, is more likely to have severe disease.
Patients with extensive **Crohn's** may have had several
surgical operations for intestinal obstruction secondary to
Stricture formation / Fistulae / Failure of medical
management. The patient with **ulcerative colitis** (UC) may
have been admitted to hospital for a severe attack of colitis
with toxic megacolon. Occasionally surgery is needed
(ileostomy and total colectomy).

PMH   Ankylosing spondylitis

FH   Increased familial incidence, but no clear-cut pattern of
inheritance

ROS   Dry, gritty red eyes / Arthralgia / Rashes

SH   Crohn's more common in smokers
UC more common in non-smokers

EXAMINATION
General appearance
         Thin / Pale / Febrile
         Erythema nodosum (50) / Arthropathy
Hands   Finger clubbing (42) rarely

Face   Conjunctivitis

Mouth   Swollen lips / Aphthous ulcers

Abdomen

Multiple laparotomy scars / Fistulae / Thickened tender mass in the right iliac fossa (RIF) (Crohn's)

Distension / Tenderness (UC)

NB: You will NOT be expected to perform a rectal examination, but you should know what you might expect to find – Oedematous skin tags / Fissuring / Ulceration / Fistulae.

INVESTIGATIONS

FBC / ESR / C-reactive protein

Albumin

LFTs (sclerosing cholangitis with UC)

Blood cultures

Stool cultures

Sigmoidoscopy (rigid / flexible) with biopsies

Small bowel enema / Meal with follow through (Crohn's)

Barium enema

Colonoscopy with biopsies

Radiolabelled white cell scan (in severe disease when radiology and endoscopy contraindicated)

TREATMENT

Maintenance

Diet (appropriate fibre intake)

5-aminosalicylic acid (5-ASA) compounds

Vitamins

Iron

Relapse

Mild   Steroids (oral / Retention enemas)

Increase dose of 5-ASA drugs

Severe   Admit to hospital

Nil by mouth

Intravenous fluids / Steroids / Anti-biotics (if septic)

Daily abdominal X-ray (colonic disease)

Surgery

Parenteral nutrition

Severe and / or continually relapsing disease may respond to immunosuppressant drugs (azathioprine) or an elemental diet.

Comment
Examiners may expect you to know the pathology of the two diseases.

Crohn's Affects any part of the gastrointestinal tract **'mouth to anus'** / Most frequently the terminal ileum

	Macro	Thickened / Narrowed bowel / Cobblestone appearance / 'Skip' lesions
	Micro	Inflammation involves ALL layers / **Granulomas**

UC Extends proximally from the rectum (occasionally involves the terminal ileum – 'backwash ileitis')

	Macro	Red, inflamed mucosa / Bleeds easily / Inflammatory polyps
	Micro	Inflammation limited to the mucosa / **crypt abscesses**

REMEMBER – **UC and colonic Crohn's are potentially pre-malignant conditions.**

Both diseases have a wide range of extra-intestinal manifestations, some of which are related to disease activity. You should know about them.

Case 24:
CHRONIC RENAL FAILURE

Think of chronic renal failure (CRF) as a multisystem disorder. Patients with CRF often spend long periods in hospital.

PC   Reason for admission (new diagnosis / Dialysis problem / Complication)

HPC   When was renal failure first diagnosed, and what were the symptoms (Lethargy / Fatigue / Anorexia / Nausea / Vomiting / Pruritus)
May have been picked up because of the discovery of Anaemia / Hypertension.
Cause of renal failure? On dialysis? If so, how long?
Continuous Ambulatory Peritoneal Dialysis (CAPD)
      How many exchanges per day (Light bags / Heavy bags)
      How many episodes of CAPD (peritonitis)
Haemodialysis   Hospital / Home
               Vascular access
               Arm / Neck / ? problems
Transplant   Functioning / Failed

PMH   Ask about disease responsible for causing renal failure if known
? Vascular disease: Angina / MI / TIAs / CVA / Claudication
Complications: Hypertension / Bone disease / Anaemia
Is the patient aware of any problem with calcium metabolism? May be awaiting parathyroidectomy.

ROS   Likely to be taking several drugs
Anti-hypertensives / Vitamin supplements / Phosphate Binders / Calcium Salts
Erythropoietin

FH   Relevant for certain causes of renal failure, eg Polycystic kidneys (39) / Alport's disease (autosomal dominant + sensorineural deafness)

SH   Likely to be unable to work
Ask about invalidity benefit etc.

? Home alterations to facilitate home haemodialysis
If CAPD, does the patient have a separate room for the
purpose?

EXAMINATION
General appearance

Anaemic / Pigmentation (36) / Excoriation (pruritus) /
Bruising
Look for arterio-venous (A-V) fistula (shunt) – usually the
forearm
Neck dialysis lines / Scars from previous insertions

CVS Hypertension / Heaving apex beat / Loud second heart
sound

Abdomen

Polycystic kidneys / Transplanted kidneys
Tenckhoff catheter – check exit site clean and healthy

CNS Fundi – hypertensive retinopathy (90)
Peripheral neuropathy (69)

Urinalysis

The patient is very likely to be anuric

INVESTIGATIONS

FBC / U&E / Calcium / Phosphate / Alkaline phosphatase
Creatinine clearance / USS
Isotope renogram / IV urography
Renal biopsy (difficult if the kidneys are small and
shrunken)

TREATMENT

Diet. All patients with CRF will have been placed on a fairly strict
'renal' diet. The essential feature is restriction of protein, potassium,
phosphate and salt. Foods which are restricted / Excluded include
chocolate, coffee, bananas, fruit drinks and dairy products.
Drugs. By the time end-stage renal failure (ESRF) occurs almost all
patients have hypertension, whatever the cause of renal
impairment, and will be on anti-hypertensives.
To prevent bone disease it is crucial to maintain normal plasma

levels of phosphate and calcium: calcium carbonate is most
frequently used (Calcichew), sometimes vitamin D.
The patient may require anti-histamines for pruritus, or anti-emetics
for nausea.
Erythropoietin, by subcutaneous injection, is used to counteract
the anaemia of CRF.

Dialysis. When the patient reaches ESRF, dialysis is implemented,
either with CAPD or with haemodialysis.
CAPD is increasingly used. Typically the patient uses four
exchanges per day, each of which is a 2 litre bag of dialysate fluid.
The glucose content, and hence the osmolality, can be varied
according to the need to remove fluid (patients will be aware of
their ideal 'dry' weight). The 'Achilles' heel' of CAPD is CAPD-
peritonitis, which usually manifests itself initially as a 'cloudy bag'.
Insulin can be added to the dialysate fluid, for those with diabetes.
Haemodialysis usually involves two to three trips each week to
hospital, each for around 6 hours. Some patients carry out their
own haemodialysis at home. There may be problems with vascular
access.

Transplantation. This requires less 'work' by the patient but
involves long-term immunosuppression which carries its own risks.
Graft rejection remains a problem, as does the lack of available
donor kidneys.

Comment
The common causes of CRF are:
Chronic glomerulonephritis
Chronic pyelonephritis
Diabetes mellitus (31)
Polycystic kidneys

Case 25:
NEPHROTIC SYNDROME

PC   Swollen ankles / legs
Frothy urine

HPC   The nephrotic syndrome comprises the classical triad of
Proteinuria / Hypoalbuminaemia / Oedema (many would
add hypercholesterolaemia).
Since three of these are essentially laboratory findings,
oedema is the only major symptom. Heavy proteinuria can
sometimes produce 'frothy urine'.
However, in less severe or very early cases, the disease
may be picked up through 'asymptomatic' proteinuria or
hyperlipidaemia.
Ask specifically about haematuria and preceding
infections.

PMH   RA / SLE / Diabetes
Known malignancy
Hodgkin's lymphoma / Myeloma (39)
TB / Osteomyelitis / Hepatitis B

FH   Familial nephritides, especially Alport's

DH   Take a careful drug history. Penicillamine / Gold (used in
the treatment of RA (37)) and captopril (used in
hypertension / Congestive cardiac failure (CCF) (13)) are
the chief culprits.
Enquire specifically about a history of atopy.

ROS
SH

EXAMINATION
General appearance
Face   Facial / Peri-orbital oedema / Xanthelasma / Butterfly rash

CVS   Hypertension
Signs of CCF

Respiratory
Pleural effusions (18) if oedema very severe

Abdomen

> May be ascites (29) / Hepatosplenomegaly (28) / Other signs of chronic liver disease (22)

CNS ? Diabetic (89) / Hypertensive retinopathy (90)
> Peripheral neuropathy (69) – may be a feature of diabetes mellitus / RA / SLE

Urinalysis

> Heavy proteinuria (± haematuria)

INVESTIGATIONS

> Urine microscopy
> 24-hour urinary protein / Creatinine clearance
> U&E / blood glucose / FBC (normochromic normocytic anaemia)
> Albumin
> Rh factor / ds-DNA / Anti-neutrophil cytoplasmic antibody / Complement
> Hepatitis B surface antigen
> Serological tests for syphilis
> Serum electrophoresis
> CXR
> Renal biopsy (unless child / long-standing diabetes / drug-induced)

TREATMENT

> Diuretics ± fluid restriction
> Salt restriction
> Angiotensin converting enzyme (ACE) inhibitors (to reduce the protein leak)
> Treat hypertension
> Treat hypercholesterolaemia
> Steroids for minimal change nephropathy and membranous nephropathy

Complication

> Renal vein thrombosis

Comment

The causes of the nephrotic syndrome can be divided into four main groups: the **glomerulonephritides** and minimal change nephropathy; **drugs; diabetes; amyloid**.

Case 26:
HEPATOMEGALY

Introduce and expose

Inspect	Distension in right Hypochondrium	
	Striae	Chronic liver disease / Obesity
	Scars	Previous tumours (? liver metastases)
		Transplant / Shunts
	Ascites	
	Stoma	Ulcerative colitis and sclerosing cholangitis / Tumours (metastasis)
Palpate	Start at RIF and move up	
	Describe liver edge	
	Smooth	Normal / Hepatitis / CCF
	Nodular	Metastasis / Cirrhosis / Tumour
	Pulsatil	Tricuspid regurgitation
	Tender	Cardiac failure / Hepatitis
Percuss	Upper and lower borders, measure size in mid-clavicular line (normal = 12 cm)	
Auscultate	Bruit Hepatocellular Carcinoma (in chronic cirrhosis). Often mistermed hepatoma. NB: it is not benign.	
	Tricuspid regurgitation	
	Arteriovenous malformation	

Don't forget the rest of the abdomen.

TEACHING POINTS
Causes

The 3 Cs	**Carcinomatosis** / hepatocellular carcinoma	
	CCF (JVP, ankle oedema) (13)	
	Cirrhosis	
Others	Fatty infiltration (alcohol)	
	Myeloproliferative disease	
	Haemochromatosis (pigmented, diabetic)	
	Lymphoproliferative disease	
	Infection (hepatitis, glandular fever, human immunodeficiency virus (HIV), hydatid)	
	Biliary obstruction	
	Infiltrates (sarcoid, amyloid)	

Comment
At the end of the examination you should be able to tell the examiner, 'There is isolated hepatomegaly with (or without) decompensation of liver function'. You should comment on any features that will lead you to a more definitive diagnosis.

Case 27:
SPLENOMEGALY

Inspect   Swelling / Bruising / Purpura
Palpate   Start in RIF and move across
               Note edge and notch
               Mass moves down with respiration
               Unable to palpate above (not ballottable)
Percuss   Dull (no bowel gas above)
               Dullness up to ninth rib / Mid-axillary line
Auscultate   Feel for any other lymph nodes – Cervical / Axillary /
               Inguinal / Epitrochlear, etc.

TEACHING POINTS
Causes

Myeloproliferative disease	**Chronic myeloid leukaemia**
	Myelofibrosis
Lymphoproliferative disease	Chronic lymphatic leukaemia
	Lymphoma
	Myelomatosis
	Acute lymphatic leukaemia
Portal hypertension	**Cirrhosis**
	Hepatic vein obstruction
Infection	**Glandular fever** / bacterial
	endocarditis
Infiltrates	Sarcoid / Amyloid

Comment
There are many more causes of spleen and liver enlargement. You should know and suggest the commoner ones as possible diagnoses.

Case 28:
HEPATOSPLENOMEGALY

You must go over all the points covered during isolated liver or spleen enlargement. It may be difficult to distinguish between massive hepatomegaly and hepatosplenomegaly. Check to see if the splenic dullness behind the ribs continues over the abdomen, if not it is more likely to be hepatomegaly alone.

TEACHING POINTS

Causes	Myeloproliferative disease
	Lymphoproliferative disease (? other lymph nodes).
	Cirrhosis with portal hypertension
	β-thalassaemia (iron deposition in skin, young)

Case 29:
ASCITES

This may appear as part of chronic liver disease or in isolation, in which case you must know the most common causes.

Inspect	Swelling / Vein distension / Everted umbilicus
Palpate	Tense / Organs may be hard to feel
	Fluctuation
	Fluid thrill
Percuss	Stony dull in flanks / Shifting dullness

TEACHING POINTS

Causes	**Cirrhosis** with portal hypertension / Chronic liver disease (22)
	Malignancy Gastrointestinal / Liver metastasis / Ovary
	Right-sided heart failure
	Nephrotic syndrome (25)
	Many others

Case 30:
RENAL MASSES

There are three main possibilities:

Unilateral enlargement
Bilateral enlargement
Transplanted kidney

The extra-abdominal signs should be noted prior to examining the abdomen.

Inspect   Scars in loin / Transplant in groin
Scars from previous CAPD catheters
A-V fistula in arm

Palpate   Bimanual palpation of mass in loin (ballottable)
Able to get above it
A transplanted kidney is found in the iliac fossa, dull to percussion (be careful with it)

Percuss   Resonant (due to bowel gas between kidney and skin)

Auscultate

Bruit Tumour / Renal artery stenosis

TEACHING POINTS

Causes   Polycystic kidneys (only one may be palpable)
Malignancy
Hydronephrosis
Hypertrophy of single or single functioning kidney
Renal cyst

Comment
Polycystic kidneys show autosomal dominant inheritance. Cysts are also found in many other organs, especially the liver, spleen and pancreas. Subarachnoid haemorrhage occurs in 5–10% of patients.

ENDOCRINE

Case 31:
DIABETES MELLITUS

Patients are frequently in hospital, either for treatment of their diabetes itself or, more commonly, for treatment of its complications.

PC   **Polyuria / Thirst / Weight loss** (insulin dependent)
Complications if longer standing (non-insulin dependent presentation)
Retinopathy Poor acuity / Blindness / Cataracts
Nephropathy Hypertension
Neuropathy
   Polyneuropathy (Sensory problems / Pain)
   Mononeuropathy (Femoral amyotrophy / Carpal tunnel)
   Autonomic neuropathy (Impotence / Diarrhoea, etc)
Vascular disease
   Peripheral / Cardiovascular / Cerebrovascular

HPC   When diagnosed / Who by / How
How does patient monitor diabetes: blood sugar (BM stix) / urinalysis
How good is control
What treatments so far (see below)
Symptoms of moniliasis
Necrobiosis lipoidica (53)

PMH May be extensive
Hypertensive

FH   Increased risk in relatives

DH   Diet / Oral hypoglycaemics
Insulin Which type: Pig / Human
                Short / Long-acting (or mixture)
                Dose / Timing
                Sites of injection (? lipohypertrophy)
                Hypoglycaemic attacks

ROS Concentrate on complications not mentioned above.

SH

EXAMINATION
General Appearance
      Well / Unwell
      Thin / Obese
CVS   Particularly BP
      Check foot pulses
Abdomen
      Injection sites

CNS   Visual acuity / Fundoscopy (89)
      Peripheral neuropathy (69)
      Absent ankle jerks / Distal sensory loss / Neuropathic
      ulcers

The diabetic foot
      Peripheral pulses
      Skin ulcers / Callous / Fungal infection / Nail care
      Neuropathy

INVESTIGATIONS
      For the patient in the exam, who is likely either to have had
      diabetes for many years or to have presented in diabetic
      ketoacidosis, the diagnosis is unlikely to be in doubt.
      However you should be aware of the strict diagnostic
      criteria.

      Glycosylated haemoglobin (HbA_{1c})
      U&E
      Cholesterol

TREATMENT
      Diet – ALL patients. The diet for a diabetic patient is no
      different from the diet considered healthy for the
      population as a whole.
      Oral hypoglycaemics
      Insulin   Human vs porcine
                   Short / Intermediate / Long-acting

Comment

Essentially there are two types of diabetes:

Insulin dependent diabetes mellitus (IDDM / Type 1)

> Young patient / Thin
> Short history / Often presents in diabetic ketoacidosis (DKA)
> Treated with insulin from time of diagnosis

Non-insulin dependent diabetes mellitus (NIDDM / Maturity onset / Type 2)

> Middle-aged / Overweight
> Often been present 'subclinically' for some time, as the degree of hyperglycaemia is usually less, and hence often presents with complications of diabetes rather than thirst, weight loss, etc.
> Treated with diet alone / Oral hypoglycaemics / Occasionally insulin later.

Case 32:
HYPERTHYROIDISM / GRAVES' DISEASE

A common disorder, and although patients are often managed as outpatients, the symptoms and signs are so classic that they often appear in medical finals.

PC   Varied
Typically weight loss / Palpitations / Anxiety / SOB

HPC   Symptoms may have been present for some time before the diagnosis is made, as they are very variable, and often non-specific. Indeed many patients are often initially given a 'psychiatric' label.
Ask specifically about Heat intolerance / Diarrhoea / Goitre / Change in appearance.

PMH   There may be a history of other auto-immune disorders (32)

FH   Frequently positive for Thyroid dysfunction / Other auto-immune disorders

DH   Is patient on treatment already β-blockers / Carbimazole?

SH

EXAMINATION
General Appearance
    Thin / Nervous / Fidgety

Hands   Sweaty palms / Tremor of the outstretched arms / Palmar erythema
Thyroid acropachy (32)

Neck   Goitre / ? Bruit (32)

Face   Exophthalmos / Lid retraction / Lid lag
Eyes (87)

CVS   Tachycardia / Atrial fibrillation (10) / Bounding pulse
Signs of heart failure (especially in the elderly)

CNS   Proximal muscle weakness (70)

Extra   Look for pre-tibial myxoedema (52)

INVESTIGATIONS
Thyroid function tests (high free T$_4$, T$_3$ / Low thyroid stimulating hormone (TSH))
Imaging techniques if goitre very large and considering surgery.
Radioisotope studies if solitary nodule

TREATMENT
Drugs   Carbimazole* for the disease
Propranolol for the symptoms
Radio-active iodine (most patients eventually become hypothyroid)
Surgery indications: Large goitre / Toxic nodule

Causes of hyperthyroidism
Graves' disease – commonest
Solitary toxic nodule (Plummer's disease – about 5%)
Toxic multinodular goitre (especially the elderly)

*Agranulocytosis can rarely occur as a side-effect (idiosyncratic) of carbimazole. Patients should be told to immediately report sore throat, fever, etc. and have their blood count checked every few weeks during initial treatment.

Comment
You need to distinguish those signs due to hyperthyroidism itself (ie simply due to an excess of circulating T_3 and T_4) from those signs which occur only in Graves' disease.

Hyperthyroidism
  Lid lag / lid retraction
  Tachycardia / Atrial fibrillation
  High output state
  Tremor
  Palmar erythema
  Proximal myopathy
Graves'
  Exophthalmos
  Pretibial myxoedema
  Acropachy

Case 33:
CUSHING'S SYNDROME

Introduce and expose

Observe	Typically	Moon face / Plethoric / Acne / Hirsute / Truncal obesity / Wasted limbs / Buffalo hump / Striae / Thin skin with increased bruising / Oral candidiasis

On recognising a patient with Cushing's syndrome tell the examiner that you would like to:

1. Measure blood pressure
2. Test for proximal weakness (70)
3. Test for glycosuria
4. Ask the patient whether they are taking steroids

TEACHING POINTS

Causes	Iatrogenic	(most often prednisolone)
	Raised ACTH	Pituitary tumour (microadenoma)
		Ectopic (small cell lung tumour (15))
	Adrenal tumour	

Comment

Remember Cushing's disease refers to one specific cause of Cushing's syndrome, ie a pituitary ACTH-secreting adenoma. By far the commonest cause of Cushing's syndrome is iatrogenic, due to the administration of long-term steroids. Hospitals are full of patients on long-term steroids. They may have obvious signs of the underlying disease, eg rheumatoid hands, loud wheeze (chronic asthma).

Case 34:
HYPOTHYROIDISM

Introduce and expose in such a way that the patient answers you.
You may hear the typical hoarse / Croaking voice

Observe	Typically	Female (middle age / Elderly)
		Overweight
	Face	Coarse facial features
		Peri-orbital puffiness
		Xanthelasma
		Loss of outer third of eyebrows
		(notoriously unreliable)
		Dry brittle hair
	Neck	? Goitre (58)

On recognising hypothyroidism tell the examiner that you would
like to ask the patient about specific features of hypothyroidism,
look for further signs and any possible predisposing factors.

Symptoms	Cold intolerance
	Lethargy
	Weight gain
	Voice change
	Constipation
Signs	Goitre (58)
	Slow relaxing tendon jerks
	Carpal tunnel syndrome (43)
	Proximal muscle weakness (70)
Predisposing factors	
	Goitre surgery
	Radioactive iodine

Case 35:
ACROMEGALY

Introduce and expose

Observe   Coarse facial features
                Prominent supra-orbital ridges
                Broad nose
                Large jaw / Prognathism (lower teeth in front of the upper (reverse bite))
                Interdental separation increased
                Large tongue
                Large hands with thick skin
                Large head (older examiners may ask about hat size)

On recognising acromegaly tell the examiner that you would like to examine:

1. The visual fields / bitemporal hemianopia (76)
   Growth hormone (GH)-secreting pituitary adenomas are usually large (cf. ACTH-secreting tumours)
2. For evidence of carpal tunnel syndrome (43)
3. The urine for glycosuria (associated diabetes – may have neuropathy etc. (69)).

Case 36:
ADDISON'S DISEASE

As this is a little more difficult you may be given a clue, eg that the patient presented with Malaise / Weight loss / Abdominal pain / Dizziness.

Introduce and expose

Observe   Female (young to middle-aged)

Thin

Pigmented skin creases / Mouth / Scars

Postural hypotension

Additional vitiligo (56)

It is very common for patients to develop more than one auto-immune condition, therefore you may be given the clue that the patient has a history of thyroid disease.

TEACHING POINTS

Other causes of pigmentation are race, haemochromatosis, ectopic, ACTH, sun tan and repeated blood transfusions.

VIVA QUESTIONS

How would you treat diabetic ketoacidosis?

Diabetic ketoacidosis is the result of insulin deficiency and may occur in the undiagnosed type I or type I diabetic patient on a suboptimal maintenance regimen or in the context of intercurrent illness that results in hormonal changes that oppose insulin action. The insulin deficiency results in elevated hepatic gluconeogenesis but peripheral tissue uptake of glucose into the tissues is poor due to the insulin deficiency. The resulting hyperglycaemia causes osmotic diuresis and dehydration. In cellular metabolism, the lack of glucose and its derivatives lead to less acetyl CoA entering the citric acid cycle; this is converted to acetoacetone. The peripheral increased oxidation of fatty acids for energy also increases the ketone burden which exceeds the ability of tissues to use them, hence a ketoacidotic state results. The metabolic acidosis and the dehydration (pre-renal failure) contribute to the attendant hyperkalaemia.

Hence, the therapy is aimed at fluid replacement and insulin replacement. These measures usually will correct the acidosis and the hyperkalaemia. Refractory severe acidosis may require sodium bicarbonate iv, and hyperkalaemia greater than or equal to 6.8 mmol/l should be tempered with calcium gluconate to prevent cardiac asystole.

Describe the use of insulin

Insulin is an anabolic hormone produced by the β-islet cells of the pancreas. It works reciprocally to glucagon to increase the storage of glucose, fatty acids and amino acids.

It increases glucose uptake into insulin sensitive cells such as muscle by upregulation of glucose transporters. Other rapid effect are amino acid and potassium uptake; intermediate effects are those protein synthesis/inhibition of degradation, activation of glucagon synthase and inhibition of gluconeogenesis; delayed effects are increasing expression of mRNA for lipogenic enzymes.

The principal clinical usage is in type I diabetes where insulin is deficient and in the acute treatment of marked hyperkalaemia;

more recently strict glycaemic control of critically ill non-diabetic patients has also been found to be of benefit.

Outline the treatment of hyperthyroidism

Thyroxine is produced by the thyroid gland and its widespread effects are due to stimulation of oxygen consumption by tissues and hence metabolic rate. It is also involved in growth, and, in mammals, fat metabolism and increased carbohydrate absorption from the intestine.

Excess results in weight loss and diarrhoea, mood disturbance, asthenia, tremor, palpitations, heat intolerance/Sweating, menstrual disorder, eye disease in Graves' and in children, tall stature.

The common causes are Graves' disease and in the elderly in particular, toxic nodular goitre; these result in overproduction in thyroxine and suppression of TSH. Rare causes include thyroid cancer, thyroiditis and choriocarcinoma.

Treatment is symptomatic with β-blockers which reduce the peripheral conversion of T_4 to (active) T_3, as well as blocking the augmentation of sympateticomimetic activity.

Anti-thyroid drugs (thionamides): these inhibit the organification of iodide and coupling of iodothyronines, hence blocking synthesis of T_4.

Radioactive iodine-[131] to ablate the thyroid tissue (not in Graves' ophthalmopathy).

Surgery when refractory to above, need for rapid euthyroid state, eg prior to planned pregnancy, and bulky goitre (cosmetic and tracheal pressure effects)

Patients may need thyroxine as iatrogenic hypothyroidism may frequently occur.

Hypothyroidism is usually due to atrophic auto-immune disease but in mountainous areas of the world, eg in South America, Central Africa and in the Himalayas it may be due to iodine deficiency. Pituitary hypothyroidism is rare. The classic clinical picture is that of slow, dry-haired, coarse skinned, deep voiced female with weight gain/constipation, cold intolerance and bradycardia. Menstrual irregularities may occur and in children short stature and poor intellectual performance.

Treatment is with T_4 100–200 micrograms daily; dose increments with TSH/T_4 monitoring, aiming for TSH in the normal range or, in the case of persistent symptoms, suppression of the TSH is aimed for.

How would you recognise a patient with Acromegaly? What questions would you ask?

Growth hormone stimulates skeletal and soft tissue growth. This causes gigantism in children if it develops prior to epiphyseal fusion, and in adults acromegaly (usually due to pituitary adenoma).

The acromegalic patient will have prominent supraorbital ridges, large nose/bridge and lips. The lower jaw will protrude causing malocclusion, and interdental separation occurs; there is macroglossia with impression of the teeth on the tongue. The hands are large with broad palms and spatulate fingers. More formal examination may reveal bitemporal visual field defect, excessive sweating, greasy skin, cardiomegaly and goitre.

One can enquire about change in facial appearance, shoe and classically, hat size; rings may now not fit; headaches and visual deterioration; sweating best correlates with disease activity. Polyuria and polydipsia may herald associated diabetes. Joint pains may be present due to chondrocalcinosis. Breathlessness may be due to cardiac failure.

What is the syndrome of inappropriate ADH secretion (SIADH)?

Inappropriate ADH activity for the patient's given level of hydration/ECF and sodium level diagnosed by demonstrating plasma osmolality < 270 mOsM/kg, Urine osmolality > 100 mOsm/kg and urine sodium > 40 mmol/l in a euvolemic patient.
Causes: Tumours of the lung and pancreas, suppurative lung disease, positive pressure ventilation, cerebral infection, tumour, inflammation or raised intracranial pressure and drugs such as phenothiazides and carbamazepine.

The cases

MUSCULOSKELETAL SYSTEM

MUSCULOSKELETAL SYSTEM
'Examine this patient's hands'

There are many diagnoses that may be picked up when are asked to look at a patient's hands. You must develop a thorough routine so as not to miss any important signs.

Introduce and expose

Observe	**General**	Cachexia
		Psoriatic skin rash
Face	Cushingoid	Rheumatoid / SLE (may have carpal tunnel syndrome)
	Exophthalmos	Thyroid acropachy (32)
	Acromegaly	CTS / Diabetic neuropathy / Thickened nerves
	Heliotrope	Dermatomyositis (48)
Hands	**Nails**	Clubbing (42)
	Splinter haemorrhages	Endocarditis (2)
	Leuconychia	Low protein states
	Nail bed infarcts	Rheumatoid (37, 40) / Systemic sclerosis (38)
	Pitting, ridging, etc.	Psoriasis
Skin	Tight	Scleroderma / CREST (44)
	Steroidal	
	Raynaud's phenomenon	
	Spider naevi	
	Gouty tophi	
	Rash of dermatomyositis	
	Palmar pigmentation	
	Tendon xanthomata	
Joints	Observe	Swelling / Deformity / Inflammation
	Palpate	Tenderness / Synovial thickening Heberden's / Osler's nodes
Nerves	Wasting	Interossei / Thenar / Hypothenar
	Weakness	First dorsal interosseous / Ulnar abductor pollicis brevis / Median
	Sensation	Pin prick / Joint position sense (JPS) / Vibration
		Differentiate between Ulnar / Median / Radial / C6 C7 C8
Function	Undo and do up buttons / write / hold cup, etc.	

Palms	Rheumatoid nodules / Dupuytren's contracture / Erythema
Wrists	Peripheral pulses
Elbows	Gouty tophi / Rheumatoid nodules
	Psoriatic plaques
	Tendon xanthomata

Case 37:
RHEUMATOID ARTHRITIS

PC   **Joint pain / Swelling** / Stiffness
        Fatigue / Malaise

HPC   Which joints affected / **Symmetrical** pattern
        Duration of 'early morning stiffness'
        Acute joint swelling (? effusion)
        Disability fasten buttons / Brush hair / Climb stairs / Walk etc.
        Symptoms of extra-articular complications

Chest pain	Pericarditis
SOB	Pleural effusion / Fibrosing alveolitis / Anaemia
Dry eyes	Painful red eyes Sjögren's / Scleritis
Neurological	Nerve entrapment / Peripheral neuropathy
Skin	Raynaud's / Nodules / Ulceration

PMH   Previous peptic ulceration (care with NSAIDs)

DH   List all treatment past and present
        Was past treatment stopped due to side effects or lack of response?
        Ask about joint injections (steroids)

FH   Family history in 5–10%

ROS

SH   In particular note the functional ability, consider helpful gadgets around the house and whether walking aids or a wheelchair are needed.

EXAMINATION
General appearance
        Pale / Tired / Unwell / Febrile / Leg ulcers / Lymphadenopathy

Hands (40)
All other joints must be examined for
> Swelling   Synovitis / Effusion
> Pain
> Erythema
> Limitation of movement

Face   Dry eyes / Scleritis / Scleromalacia

CVS   Pericardial rub

Respiratory
Pleural effusion (18) / Fibrosis (lower zones)

Abdomen
Splenomegaly (Felty's syndrome)

CNS   Carpal tunnel (43) / Peripheral neuropathy (69)

Urine   Proteinuria (Drugs / Amyloid)

INVESTIGATIONS
FBC   Anaemia (normochromic-normocytic)
   Thrombocytosis
ESR / PV   Elevated
Rheumatoid factor (80%)
   Anti-nuclear antibody (30%)
Synovial fluid analysis
X-rays   Soft-tissue swelling / Narrowing of joint space
   Erosions / Periarticular osteoporosis

TREATMENT

Drugs	You should know the most important side effects:
NSAIDs	Peptic ulcers / Iron deficiency anaemia secondary to blood loss
Sulfasalazine	Nausea / Headache / Marrow toxicity / Hepatitis / Oligospermia
Penicillamine	Metallic taste / Thrombocytopenia / Proteinuria (nephrotic syndrome)
Gold	Rash / Thrombocytopenia / Proteinuria (nephrotic syndrome)

Steroids	Weight gain / Osteoporosis / Cushing's (33)
Chloroquine	Retinopathy
Azathioprine	Nausea / Marrow toxicity / Infections, eg shingles (herpes zoster)
Methotrexate	Marrow toxicity / Pulmonary hypersensitivity / Hepatic fibrosis

Intra-articular steroids are used to manage acute exacerbations in one or two joints at a time. Joints should not be injected more than two to three times in any one year. Complications such as joint infection and skin ulceration may develop if given inappropriately or incorrectly.

Aids / Splints / Physiotherapy / general support

Comment
RA is a common disease and appears as a long case frequently. The patient in the exam with RA may have been admitted for one of three reasons:
1. Directly due to joint disease
2. Extra-articular disease
3. Complications of treatment
Hence you need to be familiar with all these aspects of the disease.

NB: the hallmark of an inflammatory arthropathy is early morning stiffness – although this can occur in osteoarthritis it is usually of short duration (half hour). Contrast the pattern of joint involvement in RA – proximal interphalangeal joints (PIPs), metacarpophalangeal joints (MCPs), wrist, elbow, shoulder, knee, ankle – with that in osteoarthritis – distal IP joints, lumbar spine, knees and hips.

Case 38:
SYSTEMIC LUPUS ERYTHEMATOSUS

A similar case to the previous one (RA) in its approach. The patients are usually young females and tend to be well informed about their condition – use their expertise.

PC	Initial presentation: When / Precipitating event?
HPC	SLE is extremely variable in its manifestation. **Arthralgia** and rash are the commonest features, but it is a truly multi-system disorder and all the following must be enquired about. (Your systemic enquiry will be exhausted during this part of the history.)
General	Weight loss / Malaise / Fever
Joints	Pain / Swelling
Skin	Facial rash / Photosensitivity / Raynaud's
Respiratory	Pleuritic chest pain / Shortness of breath
Renal	Treatment for renal failure / Dialysis
Neuro	Fits / Stroke-like episodes
PMH	Recurrent abortions (use 'miscarriages' with the patient) Previous DVT / PE History of depression (101) / Psychosis (102)
FH	
DH	Rarely certain drugs can produce an SLE-like syndrome, eg penicillamine
SH	

EXAMINATION
General appearance

Pallor / Pyrexia / Lymphadenopathy / Vasculitic rash

Hands   Raynaud's / Nail bed infarcts / Finger spindling

Face   Butterfly rash (sun sensitive)

CVS   Hypertension (related to renal disease)

Respiratory   Pleural rub / Effusion (18)

Bones and joints

Often normal (despite severe pain) / Spindling of fingers
May have severe arthritis

Neurological   Mononeuritis / Psychosis / Depression
Signs of previous CVA (thrombotic) (61)

Urine   **Proteinuria / haematuria**

INVESTIGATIONS

FBC	Anaemia of chronic disease / Leucopenia
ESR	Elevated
U&E	Renal disease
Anti-nuclear antibody	
	95%
ds-DNA	50% (but specific)
Complement	Low in active disease
Rh factor	50%
(Renal biopsy)	

TREATMENT

Chloroquine   Mild disease
Steroids   The 'mainstay' of treatment
Cyclophosphamide / Azathioprine / Serious disease (renal or cerebral involvement)
Avoid sunlight / Use sun block if photosensitive

Comment
There is a distinct overlap between the connective tissue diseases and this often confuses candidates and examiners alike. Mixed connective tissue disease (MCTD) is a useful term in cases where there are features of more than one: SLE, systemic sclerosis (44) and polymyositis (48). Investigation shows antibodies to ribonucleoprotein (part of the extractable nuclear antigen, ENA) in a speckled pattern.

Case 39:
MULTIPLE MYELOMA

PC   Bone pain
Lassitude
Infection

HPC   Bone pain, and especially back pain, is by far the commonest presenting symptom: there may be an underlying pathological fracture.
Lassitude is a prominent feature, and indeed in some is the sole complaint.
Anorexia, vomiting and depression may all occur – secondary to hypercalcaemia.
Because the symptoms tend to be rather insidious and non-specific, they have often been present for some time before the diagnosis is made.
The varied nature of the symptoms means that the patient may present to many different specialists, eg orthopaedic surgeons, general physicians, haematologists, and for those patients who present with renal failure, nephrologists.
In 10% the presentation is with **infection**. Pneumonia is characteristic, especially streptococcal.

PMH

FH   No familial incidence

DH
ROS
SH

EXAMINATION
General appearance
               Pale / Tired / Unwell
May be in obvious pain secondary to pathological fracture?
Dehydrated / ? Uraemic
Easy bruising

CVS   Very rarely heart failure secondary to hyperviscosity

Respiratory ? Pneumonia (bronchial breathing / Crackles / Effusion etc.)

Bones and joints
Examine back (erythema ab igne (54)) Vertebral collapse may cause loss of height

CNS   Peripheral neuropathy can occur

INVESTIGATIONS
Diagnostic criteria – need two or more of:
  Paraprotein in serum
  Bence Jones protein in the urine
  Plasma cells in bone marrow
FBC (normochromic, normocytic anaemia)
ESR (elevated, often to over 100)
U&Es (impaired renal function)
Hypercalcaemia (with normal alkaline phosphatase cf. bony metastasis – both up)
Skeletal survey

TREATMENT
General measures Analgesia / Rehydration
Specific   Chemotherapy / Dialysis

Comment
Multiple myeloma can affect many organ systems. The major effects of the disease can be divided into four groups:
The abnormal paraprotein itself
Hyperviscosity (raised ESR) / Abnormal platelet function / **Renal damage** / Amyloid deposition
Infiltration of the bone marrow
Anaemia / Leucopenia / Thrombocytopenia

Suppression of normal immunoglobulin
Poor humoral immunity and repeated infections
Skeletal destruction
Pathological fracture / Vertebral collapse / **Hypercalcaemia / pain**

Case 40:
RHEUMATOID HANDS

Introduce and expose

Observe		Wasting / Cushingoid
Hands		**Ask if hands are painful**
	Nails	Nail bed infarcts
	Skin	Steroidal / Raynaud's / Ulcers over nodules
	Joints	Symmetrical disease
		Soft-tissue swelling / Spindling of fingers
		Swelling / Redness / Synovitis / Especially MCP joints
		Ulnar deviation of fingers
		Swan neck deformity
		Boutonnière deformity
		Z deformity of thumb
		Subluxation of proximal phalanx
	Nerves	Wasting of small muscles of hand / Generalised weakness
		No movement if tendon ruptured
		Grip strength decreased with severity
		Change if co-existing CTS / Polyneuropathy / Ulnar entrapment at elbow
	Function	May be markedly decreased
	Extras	Nodules over tendons particularly at elbows

See also Case 8.

Case 41:
OSTEOARTHRITIS

Introduce and expose
Observe
Hands   Nails
             Skin
             Joints   Heberden's nodes (bony swelling of DIPs)
                       Bouchard's nodes (bony swelling of PIPs)
                       Squaring of hands (first carpometacarpal joint)
Nerves
Function   May be decreased

TEACHING POINTS
Primary   Middle aged women / Familial / Especially DIP
                       joint involvement
Secondary   Many causes of joint damage
                       Wear and tear / Trauma   Heavy lifting / Runners
                                                etc.
                       Disabled patients   In arm of crutch use
                       Inflammatory arthritides RA (37) / Gout (45) /
                                                Others
                       Neuropathic (Charcot) joints

Case 42:
CLUBBING

Introduce and expose

Observe	Signs of underlying disease
Hands	**Loss of angle** at the nail bed
	Increased curvature of the nail
	Fluctuation of the nail bed

When discussing the possible underlying causes you must look for any pointers about the diagnosis in that patient.

TEACHING POINTS

Causes:

Lung	Carcinoma of the bronchus	Tar stains / Cachexia
	Fibrosing alveolitis	Dyspnoea
	Bronchiectasis	Sputum pot
	Mesothelioma	
Bowel	Cirrhosis	Signs of liver disease
	Inflammatory bowel disease	Wasted
Heart	Endocarditis	Splinter haemorrhages
	Cyanotic congenital heart disease	Down's syndrome
	Myxoma	
Thyroid	Acropachy	Exophthalmos / Goitre
Hereditary	Idiopathic	

Case 43:
ULNAR / MEDIAN / T1 LESIONS

	Ulnar	Median	T1
Observe	Clawing fourth and fifth fingers		
Wasted muscles	Hypothenar interossei	Thenar	All small muscles
Weakness	Add/abduction of fingers	Abductor pollicis brevis	All
Sensory Loss	Medial 1.5 digits	Lateral 3.5 digits	Medial forearm
Extras	Deformed elbow Rheumatoid	Tinel's sign at wrist over carpal tunnel Scar at wrist	Neck Lymphadeno-pathy Ipsilateral Horner's

TEACHING POINTS
Causes
The median and ulnar nerves may be damaged anywhere along their course due to trauma. Common sites of entrapment are: the carpal tunnel (median nerve), the elbow in patients with rheumatoid arthritis (median and / or ulnar nerves). The nerves can of course be individually affected by a mononeuropathy.

T1 root lesions may be due to damage anywhere along its course:
Cord (especially bilateral)	Syringomyelia (84) / Tumour
Root	Cervical spondylosis
Plexus	Pancoast tumour (assn. Horner's syndrome (61)) / Cachexia etc)

Comment
A radial nerve lesion is less common. The clinical features are sensory loss over the lateral dorsum of the hand and adjacent forearm, and motor weakness involving the extensors of the wrist and fingers, supinator and the extensor carpi radialis, giving **wrist drop**.

99

Case 44:
SCLERODERMA / CREST

Although rare in clinical practice, this is commonly seen in examinations.

Introduce and expose

Observe	General	(Signs of mixed connective tissue disease (39))
	Face	Tight skin around mouth / Telangiectasia / Dry eyes
Hands	Skin	Tight / Shiny / Spindle shaped fingers / Calcinosis / Raynaud's / Pulp infarcts / Autoamputation
	Nails	Nail bed infarcts
	Joints	Swollen
	Nerves	Usually none / Carpal tunnel / Proximal muscle weakness (43)
	Function	May be severely restricted
Arms		Skin changes may occur over much of the body surface.

TEACHING POINTS

Systemic sclerosis is a multisystem disease and although the skin changes are the most obvious manifestation, joint, gastrointestinal, renal and cardiorespiratory complications are the main causes of morbidity and mortality.

Comment

One of the most troublesome features is coldness. The patient may have battery heated gloves.

Case 45:
GOUT

TOPHACEOUS GOUT
Introduce and expose

Observe	Obesity / Ruddy 'Boozer's' face	
Hands	Nails	
	Skin	Thin or ulcerated over tophi (subcutaneous yellow / white nodules)
	Joints	**Asymmetrical** swelling of small joints
		Tophi over joints
	Nerves	Associated carpal tunnel syndrome (43)
Elbows	Tophi	
Function	May be decreased depending on severity	
Extras	Look for tophi on ear	
	Similar picture on the feet	

TEACHING POINTS

Differential diagnosis at elbow	Rheumatoid nodules
Complications	Renal stones
	Carpal tunnel syndrome

Comment
Occasionally there is gross deformity of the joints due to tophus formation and joint margin erosions. Uric acid crystals are needle shaped and negatively birefringent. Treatment of the acute attack is with NSAIDs and of the chronic condition with allopurinol.

GOUT – SINGLE JOINT
You may be asked to comment on a single inflamed joint (Red / Tender / Swollen).
The hallux is the joint most often affected.

TEACHING POINTS

Precipitating factors	Drugs: Aspirin / Diuretics / Allopurinol
	Stress / Surgery
	Exercise

Case 46:
PAGET'S DISEASE

You will be asked to 'Look at this patient's face' (or legs).

FACE
Introduce and expose
Observe   Increased size of skull
              Hearing aid

There may be other cranial nerve lesions due to compression as
they leave through the many skull foramina
              Poor vision / Optic atrophy (angioid streaks seen on
              funduscopy)
              VIth nerve palsy

LEGS
Introduce and expose
Observe   Bowing of tibia (anteriorly)
                Unilateral
Palpate   Warmth (high blood flow)
Auscultate   Bruit

TEACHING POINTS
Complications
                Bone pain / Headache
                Fractures
                Poor mobility
                Nerve / Spinal cord compression
                Hypercalcaemia
                Sarcomatous change
                High output cardiac failure (rare)

Comment
The differential diagnosis is of syphilitic sabre tibia and rickets.
Rickets is usually bilateral and syphilis is rare, offer to look for other
associated signs (63).

Case 47:
ANKYLOSING SPONDYLITIS

There is often a hint in the examiner's instruction: you might be asked to examine the neck, to watch the patient walk or to watch the patient look at the ceiling.

Observe   Young / Middle-aged male

Posture   'Question-mark' posture: loss of lumbar lordosis, kyphosis and extension of cervical spine, in order for the patient to look straight ahead.
Protuberant abdomen.

Neck   When asked to turn the head to the side, the whole body turns – the spine is rigid, with little movement.

TEACHING POINTS
Ankylosing spondylitis has a strong association with HLA-B27.
Most patients present with low back pain.
There are a number of recognised complications, eg iritis, apical fibrosis.

VIVA QUESTIONS

How would you monitor Rheumatoid arthritis?

RA is a systemic auto-immune disorder of unknown aetiology characterised by symmetrical small > large joint arthritis, pain, early morning stiffness, joint swelling and limitation of function with destructive joint disease and ankylosis.

Close clinical monitoring of the patient is required as regards symptoms/Signs of active synovitis and acquisition of functional impairment due to the destructive arthritis; this is supplemented by hand and foot X-rays to look for erosive disease evolution and serological markers of inflammation and rheumatoid factor titres.

Describe the rash that you may see in SLE?

SLE is a chronic episodic disease affecting all races but with a predisposition for women and black Americans. Impaired cellular immunity is seen with exaggerated humoral immunity with production of autoantibodies to nuclear elements.

A photosensitive erythematous rash in a butterfly distribution on the face is the classic rash seen in SLE.

What autoantibodies do you see in SLE?

Anti-nuclear antibodies non specific and present in 95%; antibodies to ds-DNA are specific but only present in 75%.

What X-ray changes may you see in multiple myeloma? What are the other cardinal feature?

Myeloma is a plasma cell dyscrasia caused a monoclonal expansion of plasma cells that secrete monoclonal immunoglobin.

The characteristic appearance on X-ray is that of lytic lesions – rounded translucencies caused by osteoclast activating factor being produced by the infiltrating myeloma cells. Radiodense expanded areas may occur due to myeloma cell infiltration called plasmacytomas. Osteopenia due to osteoporosis may also be due to myeloma and predispose to fractures especially of the vertebrae.

The cardinal clinical features are bone pain (vertebral fractures may lead to loss of height and spinal cord / Spinal root compression), symptomatic anaemia, immuneparesis with recurrent infection, renal failure (due to hypercalcaemia, dehydration, hyperuricaemia, paraprotein or amyloidosis) and bleeding due to thrombocytopenia.

What are Osler's nodes and who was Osler?

Osler's nodes are the painful indurated areas on the pads of the fingers seen in bacterial endocarditis.

Sir William Osler was a Canadian-born physician, who as a pathologist wrote the classical papers on hereditary telangiectasia (he lends his name to the eponym, Osler–Weber–Rendu), SLE and polycythaemia rubra vera. He was also Professor of Medicine at Oxford University.

What do you think of when you see a patient with clubbing?

Clubbing is the increased curvature of the nails with obliteration of the angle of the nail. Mechanisms include increased blood flow in the limbs in right to left shunt, hence bypassing the lungs' ability to inactivate systemic vasodilators; vagal mediation (reversal of clubbing by vagotomy in bronchogenic carcinoma); increased growth hormone states, and activated platelets preferentially streaming into the capillary beds of the fingers with release of platelet derived growth factor, causing increased permeability and fibroblast proliferation and hyperplasia.
Causes can be grouped:
Chest – carcinoma, fibrosing alveolitis, suppurative lung disease.
Heart – infective endocarditis, cyanotic heart disease.
Gastrointestinal – cirrhosis, inflammatory bowel disease. Thyroid acropathy and acromegaly.

How would you treat acute gout?

Gout is a disorder of purine metabolism. The hyperuricaemia is due to either overproduction or under-excretion of uric acid. This can be primary as in enzyme abnormality or renal tubular transport defect, or secondary such as due to increased production in lymphoproliferative disorders and reduced excretion due to thiazides. The uric acid is deposited in the joints and other tissues.

The acute arthritis usually affects the big toe. Treatment is with NSAIDs for pain. Steroid may confer dramatic relief in refractory cases. Colchicine is also used where NSAIDs have failed and inhibits macrophage migration and phagocytosis of uric acid. Allopurinol may worsen acute gout. It confers prophylaxis by inhibiting xanthine oxidase, hence reducing the uric acid pool.

What are the X-ray features of ankylosing spondylitis?

Ankylosing spondylitis is a chronic inflammatory disorder which predominantly affects the sacroiliac joints and has a strong association with HLA-B27. The classic X-ray finding is that of sacroiliitis as evidenced by erosions and sclerosis. Later marginal syndesmophytes develop in the lumbosacral spine and 'squaring' of the vertebral body appearance due to calcification of the interspinous ligaments gives the radiological 'bamboo spine'.

An asymmetrical large joint arthritis and enthesopathy (particularly Achilles) can occur (case 47).

Describe the typical symptoms of carpal tunnel syndrome

Compression of the median nerve at the wrist causes numbness, paraesthesia and pain in the distribution of the median nerve in the hand, although often the patient complains of whole hand numbness. Typically the symptoms are worse at night, waking the patient from sleep and vigorous hand shaking behaviour on part of the patient is exercised to afford relief. As progression occurs, the patient begins to drop things and lose manual dexterity. The evolution of the pain to sensory loss and wasting of the thenar eminence herald end-stage entrapment.

SKIN

SKIN
'Look at this patient's rash'

Skin diseases often cause confusion amongst students, mainly due to the extra terms that dermatologists use to describe lesions. To 'demystify' dermatology we think it is useful to describe a skin lesion as any surgical lump (this is something that should be second nature by the time of finals) and then use specific terms when needed.

The features of a lump that should be described are given below; some specific dermatological terms are also given. It is not necessary to use these all the time but when used appropriately it shows a greater understanding on your part.

Colour	Erythema	Increased perfusion
Shape	Plaque	Flat topped disc
	Macule	Flat area of discoloration
Size	Papule	< 1 cm of elevated skin
	Nodule	>1 cm palpable mass
Surface	Vesicle	Blister < 5 mm
	Bulla	Blister > 5 mm
	Pustule	Blister containing pus
	Scale	Flaky keratin
	Crust	Dried exudate
Site	Exact position if localised	
	? Flexor or extensor if generalised	

Edge

In the case of an ulcer you should describe the edge / base / depth / discharge / Surrounding tissues.

To practise describing skin lesions, look at a colour atlas of dermatology and go through how you would present a similar case if you saw it in the exam.

There are only a finite number of skin lesions and those likely to come up as a short case are even fewer. Systemic diseases that have cutaneous manifestations or dermatological conditions that have systemic complications are the commonest short cases and you should be aware of these. Primary dermatological diseases are unlikely to come up unless a patient happens to have co-existing eczema.

You should be familiar with the following rashes / Skin lesions and their systemic diseases:

Skin sign	Disease
Dermatitis herpetiformis	Coeliac disease
Lupus pernio/nodules	Sarcoidosis
Necrobiosis lipoidica (53)	Diabetes
Pre-tibial myxoedema (52)	Graves' disease
Erythema nodosum (50)	Many
Hereditary haemorrhagic telangiectasia (57)	Blood loss (GI/lung)
Acanthosis nigricans	Malignancy/diabetes/Cushing's
Vitiligo (56)	Many
Lupus	Discoid/systemic (38)
Neurofibromatosis (51)	Many systemic complications
Adenoma sebaceum etc.	Tuberose sclerosis (epilepsy/low IQ)
Port wine stain	Sturge–Weber (epilepsy)
Erythema multiforme (55)	Infections/drugs
Purpura	Haematological problems
Erythema ab igne (54)	Pain ? Cause

Tendon xanthomata / Xanthelasma / Eruptive xanthomata / Palmar xanthomata are associated with different hyperlipidaemias. Be sure to know which skin lesion is which.

Other common skin problems include

Ulcers Venous

       Ischaemic   Rheumatoid / Sickle / Vascular
                        insufficiency

       Neuropathic

Eczema

Psoriasis   (49)

Lichen planus   Itchy wrists / Wickham's striae in mouth

Pityriasis rosea Oval lesions on trunk / Herald patch

Pityriasis versicolor (56)

Rosacea   Facial papules / Pustules / Telangiectasia
                 Eye blepharitis / Conjunctivitis / Iritis

Shingles   Herpes zoster (common)
                 Erythematous rash over dermatome / Associated
                 pain

Case 48:
DERMATOMYOSITIS POLYMYOSITIS

Introduce and expose

Observe	Cachexia	
Face	Heliotrope rash around eyes with mild oedema	
Hands	Nails	Rash around nail bed
	Skin	Purple rash over knuckles (extensor surface of elbows and knees)
		Raynaud's phenomenon
Other	Proximal muscle weakness and muscle tenderness	

TEACHING POINTS
M:F 2:1
Malignancy 30% age 30, 40% age 40, 50% age 50, etc.
Overlap with mixed connective tissue disease (44)

Investigation Serum creatine kinase and ESR increased
EMG changes (small, short motor unit potentials)
Muscle biopsy

Treatment Oral steroids

Comments
Polymyositis is a similar condition which includes the muscle
weakness and tenderness but without the skin changes (48).

Case 49:
PSORIASIS

You may come across this either when asked to examine the hands or to comment on the rash. Invariably, one will lead on to the other.

Introduce and expose

Observe		Generalised skin changes
Hands	**Nails**	Pitting / Ridging / Onycholysis / Hyperkeratosis / Discoloration
	Skin	Plaques
		Sausage-shaped fingers
	Joints	Distal interphalangeal joint swelling
		Rheumatoid pattern (symmetrical small joint swelling)
		Arthritis mutilans (telescoping of phalanges)
		Monarthritis of larger joints
		Ankylosing spondylitis / Sacroiliitis type
	Rash	Salmon pink plaques / Silver white scales

Look or ask to see extensor surfaces / Scalp / Navel / Natal cleft

---

Comment

There are several types of skin lesion – chronic plaques, guttate, pustular and erythrodermic. Many drugs can exacerbate the condition including alcohol/β-blockers/NSAIDs/lithium.

Case 50:
ERYTHEMA NODOSUM

Site   Shins (occasionally thighs)
Description   Tender / Red / Raised lesions 2–6 cm in diameter

Causes   Sarcoidosis
             Streptococcal infection
             Drugs (sulphonamides / Penicillin / oral
             contraceptive)
             Inflammatory bowel disease
             Primary TB
             Pregnancy
             Rheumatic fever
             Many others

Case 51:
NEUROFIBROMATOSIS

Introduce and expose

Observe	Skin lesions	Café-au-lait spots (> 5)
		Axillary freckling
		Subcutaneous
		Neurofibromata
		Mollusca fibrosa (pink cutaneous fibromas)
		Plexiform neuroma
	Skeletal	Kyphoscoliosis (50%)

There may be very, very many skin lesions and gross neurofibromatosis can be quite disfiguring.

Eyes	Visual acuity may be decreased due to optic glioma
	Fundal changes
	Iris nodules (of Lisch) difficult to see
Hearing	Decreased with acoustic neuroma
BP	Raised if **renal artery stenosis** (intimal hyperplasia) or more rarely phaeochromocytoma

TEACHING POINTS
Neurological complications
   Intracranial / Intraspinal / Peripheral nerve tumours
   All types of tumour may occur (glioma / Neuroma / Meningioma / Neurofibroma – 'a tumour soup')
   The signs will be dependent on the location of the tumour.

Comment
There are two types of neurofibromatosis, both show autosomal dominant inheritance. Positive family history in 50%.
Type I   As described above
         Von Recklinghausen's disease / Chromosome 17.

Type II Bilateral VIIIth nerve tumours / No skin or skeletal lesions / Intracranial and intraspinal tumours also common / Chromosome 22.

Case 52:
PRE-TIBIAL MYXOEDEMA

Site   Shins (± feet)

Description   Raised / Purple-red lesions with 'orange peel'
                  appearance
                  If severe, skin thickened with non-pitting oedema

Cause   Graves' disease (32)

NB: Pre-tibial myxoedema usually develops after the
hyperthyroidism has been treated.
Look for exophthalmos or a thyroidectomy scar.

Case 53:
NECROBIOSIS LIPOIDICA

Site   Shins (occasionally arms)

Description   Shiny yellow plaques with waxy centre
                  Brown-red margins and nearby telangiectasias

Cause   **Diabetes mellitus** (31)
                  Look for tell-tale signs on patient's bedside locker –
                  BM stix / Sugar-free juice / Diabetic chocolate etc.

Case 54:
ERYTHEMA AB IGNE

Site   Commonly shins, or lateral aspect of one leg, from
                  sitting next to the fire. Also low back, from exposure
                  to hot water bottle.

Description   Pigmented / Erythematous reticular discoloration

Causes   Exposure to excessive heat, therefore: chronic pain /
                  Myeloma (39). Intolerance of cold (? hypothyroid)

Case 55:
ERYTHEMA MULTIFORME

Site	Limbs and trunk
	Classically, backs of hands, forearms, feet and toes

Description Red papules with central pallor – 'target lesions'
Bullae can develop within the lesions

Causes Unknown (50%)

Infection	Herpes simplex / Mycoplasma Pneumonia
Drugs	Sulphonamides / Penicillin
Connective tissue diseases	
Neoplasia	

Comment

Stevens–Johnson syndrome is a severe form, with widespread bullous eruptions and orogenital ulceration. It is potentially life-threatening.

Case 56:
VITILIGO PITYRIASIS

Site	Anywhere
	Often hands, face and neck, dorsum of feet

Description	Symmetrical patches of depigmentation with hyperpigmented borders
Causes	Vitiligo is associated with organ specific auto-immune diseases of which more than one may be present in an individual. Look for alopecia and ask for a family history of vitiligo or associated diseases.

Thyroid disease
Pernicious anaemia
Addison's disease   (36)
Diabetes mellitus   (31)
Alopecia areata
Chronic active hepatitis
Primary biliary cirrhosis
Fibrosing alveolitis   (19)

PITYRIASIS VERSICOLOR
This is a skin infection caused by the yeast Pityrosporum orbiculare (Malassezia furfur) which may look like vitiligo. It is noticed especially when the patient has been sunbathing, with white patches on the tanned skin, but pale brown patches on non-exposed areas.

Case 57:
HEREDITARY HAEMORRHAGIC TELANGIECTASIA

Osler–Weber–Rendu syndrome

This case is very often introduced to the candidate by telling them that the patient presented with anaemia and / or that the patient has a daughter / Son / parent with the same problem (**autosomal dominant**).

Introduce and expose

Observe   **Pale**   Blood loss (iron deficiency anaemia)

Lung – haemoptysis (bronchiectasis)

Gut – haematemesis

Telangiectasias   Face / Around the mouth / On tongue and the undersurface of the tongue

VIVA QUESTIONS

What are the treatments for psoriasis?

Psoriasis is a chronic inflammatory skin disorder of unknown cause. Well-demarcated salmon-pink plaques with silvery scales are found on extensor areas, scalp, naval and natal cleft.
Symptomatic treatment is directed towards the pruritus and skin dryness. This can be in the form of topical emollients. Scaling can be reduced by topical keratolytics.

Topical treatment is with coal tar, steroids and calcipotriol (vitamin D_3 increases differentiation of cell and reduced rash and scale).

Systemic therapies are with photochemotherapy with PUVA (psoralens and UVA) which is successful at clearing and delaying recurrence in chronic disease.

Etretinate (vitamin A derivative) and the folate antagonist methotrexate are used in severe disease unresponsive to other therapies. Steroids, hydroxyurea, colchicine and ciclosporin may also be helpful.

What types of arthritis may you see in psoriasis?

The inflammatory arthritis has a predilection for the distal interphalangeal joints of the hands but four variations are seen; an asymmetrical arthritis, symmetrical arthritis – rheumatoid-like, sacroiliitis and arthritis mutilans which there is resorption of the phalanges and 'telescoping' of the digits (case 49).

NECK

NECK
'Examine this patient's neck'

This command indicates one of three possibilities:
Abnormal JVP
Cervical lymphadenopathy
Goitre ± abnormal thyroid status

If the patient is sitting on a chair that you can get behind and / or there is a glass of water nearby, it is most likely to be a goitre and less likely to be an abnormal JVP. If the patient is on a bed and is able to lean back the opposite is true. This is a difficult case. However, if you are methodical you will not miss anything.

Introduce and expose

Observe	**General**	Thyroid eyes – exophthalmos / lid retraction
		Glass of water nearby – goitre
		Dyspnoea – cor pulmonale (right heart failure)
		Wasting – malignancy / lymphadenopathy
Inspect	**Neck**	Obvious goitre? Yes – Go on to Case 58
		No – Go on to Case 59

Case 58:
GOITRE

Palpate the mass as for any lump
? Single nodule / Multinodular / Diffusely enlarged
Ask the patient to swallow (after they have taken a sip of water and held it in their mouth).
A goitre should move up.
Palpate for any associated lymphadenopathy.

Percuss over the top of the manubrium / Dullness may indicate a retrosternal thyroid.

Auscultate over the thyroid for a bruit.

Ask the examiner if you could test the thyroid status.
Also ask to look for eye signs.

Comment
To revise the thyroid fully you must look at the four cases 32 / 34 / 52 / 58.

Case 59:
LYMPHADENOPATHY

Inspect   Neck   Obvious raised JVP?   Yes – Go to Case 60
                                                No – Carry on

Ask patient to sit forward

Palpate each of the neck areas in turn (**from behind**).
Describe the lump or lumps as you would any 'surgical lump':
Site / Shape / Surface etc.

The most common diagnoses are:
1. Reactive (infection)
2. Neoplastic metastases
3. Lymphoma
4. Tuberculosis

If no goitre and no lymphadenopathy look carefully for the JVP.

Case 60:
JUGULAR VENOUS PRESSURE

It is almost impossible to describe in print the difficult job of assessing the JVP. We strongly advise you to arrange bedside teaching before the exam, which is by far the best way to understand what is going on.

Lean the patient back at 45 degrees
Look for raised JVP (may be above ear)
    Measure height above the sternal angle
    If not seen gently press abdomen (remember to ask patient first)
    Time pulsation against opposite carotid pulse

Big systolic V wave	CCF / Tricuspid regurgitation
Big diastolic A wave	Pulmonary hypertension
	Pulmonary / Tricuspid stenosis
	Heart block (unlikely in exams)

Non-pulsatile SVCO (20) / Excessively high CCF (13)

VIVA QUESTIONS

What diagnosis would you consider in a patient with persistent generalised lymphadenopathy – (1) a 25-year-old and (2) a 65-year-old.

The causes of generalised lymphadenopathy are lymphoma, chronic lymphoid leukaemia (CLL), acute leukaemia, Epstein–Barr virus (EBV) infection, human immunodeficiency virus (HIV) infection, toxoplasmosis, TB, secondary syphilis, brucellosis, SLE, RA, sarcoid and drugs, eg phenytoin.

A 25- and 65-year-old share the risk of lymphoma (also most common cause) but the former is more likely to have EBV, HIV and given the resurgence, syphilis. CLL is a disorder of the over-50s and acute leukaemias are statistically more common in this age group.

NEUROLOGY

NERVOUS SYSTEM
'Examine this patient's arms'

Introduce and expose

Observe	Wasting (especially small muscles of hand)
	Fasciculation

Arms outstretched

	Pyramidal drift
	Winging of scapula
Tone	With the patient relaxed passively flex and extend the elbow, feel for a supinator catch and test for cogwheeling at the wrist.
Power	Test each in turn, always comparing the two sides

	Root value
Shoulder abduction	C5
Elbow flexion	C6
Elbow extension	C7
Wrist flexion	C7, C8
Wrist extension	C6, C7
Finger extension	C7
Finger spread	T1 (ulnar)
Thumb abduction	T1 (median)

Reflexes	Demonstrate the biceps (C5), supinator (C6) and triceps (C7) jerks. Remember to use reinforcement before pronouncing a reflex absent. If reflexes brisk look for Finger flexion jerks and Hoffman's sign
Sensation	Light touch and pinprick, touch each arm once in dermatomes C4–T2. Vibration at distal phalanx: if absent, Wrist / Elbow / Shoulder.
	Joint position sense (JPS) – test using distal phalanx of one finger on each side. If absent, Wrist / Elbow.
Co-ordination	Test for finger–nose inco-ordination (Hold your finger at arm's length / No need to move finger)

NERVOUS SYSTEM
'Examine this patient's legs'

Introduce and expose

Observe	Wasting / Fasciculation / Pes cavus / Walking aids / Wheelchair
	Foot drop splint

Tone	With patient relaxed, gently roll the leg – the ankle should 'flop'
	Flex the knee quickly – feel for a 'catch'
Clonus	Check for ankle patellar clonus

Power   Test each in turn, always comparing the two sides

Activity	Root value	Main muscle
Hip flexion	L1, L2	Iliopsoas
Hip extension	S1	Glutei
Knee flexion	L5, S1	Hamstrings
Knee extension	L3, L4	Quadriceps femoris
Ankle dorsiflexion	L4, L5	Tibialis anterior
Ankle plantar flexion	S1	Gastrocnemius

Reflexes	Knee jerk (L3 / L4)
	Ankle jerk (S1)
	Remember to use reinforcement before deciding a reflex is absent
	Plantar responses (use an orange stick)

Sensation	Light touch (LT) / Pinprick (PP)
	Touch each leg once in dermatomes L2–S2.
	Light touch sensation is not always very helpful and sometimes only confuses things, make sure that you are confident in detecting the main patterns of sensory (especially PP) loss (see below).
	Vibration at medial malleoli
	If absent, knee / Iliac crest / Sternum
	JPS – use big toe on each side
	If absent ankle / knee

Hot and cold sensations are carried in the same tracts as PP, testing is therefore omitted.
Diagnoses
Distal polyneuropathy (glove / Stocking PP > LT)
Dermatomal root lesion (PP ? LT)
Spinothalamic loss (PP but not JPS / Vibration)
Dorsal column loss (JPS / Vibration not PP)

Co-ordination
Test for heel–shin ataxia

At this stage tell the examiner 'At this stage I would usually go on to examine the back for scars, assess the gait and test for Romberg's sign'. Hopefully they will stop you and ask you to present your findings.

Gait (74)   Ask the patient to walk a short way, turn around and walk back. Be sure to note
Posture / Arm swing / Step size and equality / Circumduction / Ataxia

Romberg's sign
Positive if patient falls when eyes are closed. This implies proprioceptive loss.

NERVOUS SYSTEM
'Examine this patient's cranial nerves'

It is not usual practice to expect a candidate to examine all 12 nerves and to look at the fundi on one request. Rather, you will be asked to look at an already dilated fundus, look at the eyes (meaning IInd, IIIrd, IVth and VIth nerves) or examine the lower cranial nerves (meaning Vth–XIIth but not the VIth).
However, be prepared to start at the top and work down. You must practise cranial nerve examination many times.

I   Ask the patient 'Have you noticed any problems with your sense of taste or your ability to smell things?' If the answer is yes tell the examiner you would usually go on to test these sensations formally and check to see if the patient can breathe through each nostril.

Eyes   **Observe** Ptosis: IIIrd / Sympathetic / Myasthenia
                        Squint (88):   Congenital / Acquired
                        Exophthalmos: Thyroid ophthalmoplegia

II   **Acuity** – remember that visual acuity is the single most important function of vision, without it a person is blind. Ask, 'Do you wear glasses or contact lenses?' If yes, ask them to put them on and tell the examiner 'At this stage I usually test the visual acuity formally with a Snellen chart at 6 m.' He may then tell you the acuity; if not, test it with a pocket Snellen chart held at the appropriate distance (this looks more impressive than picking up the nearest newspaper). It is important to look very confident when testing acuity so practise it until you do.
        Fields – Test these against your own with a red hat pin. Do not forget to test for a central scotoma. Practise looking good at this as well, it is very easy to see whether a candidate has any idea of what he or she is doing.
        Pupils – Have a bright pen torch to test direct response and consensual response. Test the response to accommodation by asking the patient to look at the far side of the room and then at your finger which should be held 10 cm away from the patient's nose. Make sure you are in a position to see the pupillary response.

The cases

Fundi – Leave this until the end.
Look at the discs followed by the rest of the fundus in a consistent order. (If you are told that the patient has decreased acuity while being handed an ophthalmoscope look at the macular area after the disc as this is where the pathology is most likely to be.)
Usually fundal examination is considered as a separate case.

III, IV, VI

Ask the patient to follow your pen torch and to tell you if he sees double. Hold it vertically when testing the medial and lateral recti and horizontally when testing the other muscles.
Comment on which muscles are not working. If it is not obvious when the patient complains of diplopia, cover up one eye and ask which image disappears (the outermost image is from the affected eye, ie the one that has not moved).
If nystagmus is present describe which eye is affected the most and the direction the fast phase is in (82 / 83).

V

Motor – Ask the patient to open his mouth (pterygoids). Ask the patient to clench his teeth together (masseters / Temporalis)
Sensory – Check sensitivity to pin and touch over the three divisions.
Tell the examiner 'At this stage I would usually test the corneal reflex'. It is unlikely that you will be expected to do this but you should know that the afferent limb of the reflex is trigeminal and the efferent limb is through the facial nerve to the orbicularis oculi muscles.

VII

Assess the patient's facial movements by asking him to close his eyes tightly, raise his eyebrows and show his teeth.

VIII

Ask the patient if he has any problem hearing with either ear. Rub the hair near his ear between your finger and thumb. Tuning fork tests may be needed if there is decreased hearing. Otoscopy is not expected but should be offered if there is a suggestion of a conductive defect. It is important to test hearing in any patient who has a nearby cranial nerve lesion (V/VII/IX/X) as a tumour compressing more than one nerve may be the underlying problem (95).

IX, X   Watch for palatal movement when the patient is saying 'Ahh'. The side that does not move is the abnormal one. Do not get into discussions of uvula movements, these only confuse the matter.
Tell the examiner 'At this stage I would normally test the gag reflex in order to assess sensation.' You won't usually be expected to do this.

XII   Look at the tongue inside the mouth for wasting and fasciculation (lower motor neurone (LMN) signs) and then ask the patient to move it. A spastic tongue will not be wasted but will move slowly.

XI   Ask the patient to shrug his shoulders and then to turn his head from one side to the other while you palpate the sternomastoid muscles.

Case 61:
STROKE

PC Weakness / Collapse / Visual disturbance / Dizziness / Speech problems / Sensory upset / Headache

HPC

Onset	**Sudden**
Course	Static / Resolving
History	Previous CVA / TIAs
	Amaurosis fugax
	Transient sensory / Motor problems
Risk factors	**Smoking**
	Hypertension
	Diabetes
	Hyperlipidaemia

Right or left-handed?

PMH Angina / Myocardial infarction / Rheumatic heart disease (atrial fibrillation)
Claudication

FH Increased vascular disease in family members

DH Anti-hypertensive medication
Aspirin
Warfarin (may be the cause if haemorrhagic stroke)

ROS Ask about complications
   Weight loss / Constipation / Bladder symptoms
   Shoulder subluxation / Pneumonia (aspiration)

SH

Home	House type / Ground floor / Modifications (stair lift / bath seat / downstairs commode)
	Dependants / Carers (relatives / friends / home helps, etc.)
Allowances	
Mobility	Chair / Sticks / Zimmer

EXAMINATION
General appearance
    Plethoric / Malar flush

CVS   Atrial fibrillation (10) / Heart murmurs
        BP and signs of hypertensive heart disease
        Carotid bruits

CNS   Dysphasia (100) / Dysarthria / Apraxia / Sensory / Visual
        inattention

Cranials Homonymous hemianopia (75)
        Facial weakness (upper motor neurone (UMN) lesion) (94)
        Pseudobulbar palsy (99)

Limbs   Hemiparesis
        UMN signs on one side ± sensory loss

INVESTIGATIONS
    FBC (polycythaemia) / ESR
    Glucose
    ECG
    CXR
    Cholesterol
    CT brain
    Carotid Doppler ultrasound (even if no carotid bruits)
    Echocardiogram if murmur

TREATMENT
    Acute   Aspirin keep hydrated / Good nursing care / Do not treat initial hypertension
    In-patient   Screen for risk factors / Nutrition / Aspirin Physiotherapy / occupational therapy

Comment

Definition: a stroke is a sudden neurological deficit of vascular origin lasting longer than 24 hours.

Causes   Haemorrhage 15%   (subarachnoid haemorrhage 5% / Intracerebral 10%)

Infarction 85%   (thrombotic / Embolic (from the heart or great vessels)

Clinical divisions

Carotid circulation

Hemiparesis
Homonymous Hemianopia
Dysphasia / Neglect
Hemisensory loss

Vertebrobasilar

Ipsilateral cranial nerve lesion /
Contralateral Hemiparesis
Cerebellar / Brainstem Strokes

Case 62:
MULTIPLE SCLEROSIS

The patient is often young.

PC   Details of reasons for present admission, eg difficulty walking, loss of balance, double vision, bladder symptoms, respite.

HPC   When and how did patient first present
Course of illness to date – **Relapsing / Remitting v Chronic progressive**. If relapsing Number / Frequency / Nature of relapses
Ascertain level of patient's disability, if any, in their 'steady state'
Enquire carefully about bladder symptoms – urgency / Urge incontinence. Recurrent UTIs ? Intermittent self-catheterisation / Urosheath / Indwelling catheter
It may be appropriate to ask male patients about impotence
Fatigue is very common

PMH

FH   No clear-cut pattern of inheritance: 5–15 × risk if first degree relative affected

DH   Baclofen for spasticity / Anti-cholinergics for urge incontinence
iv steroids for recent relapse

SH   This section of the history needs to be very thorough.
Able to work / Invalidity benefit / Other allowance
Ambulant / Wheelchair / Able to transfer
Carer / District nurses / Home help

EXAMINATION
Multiple sclerosis (MS), by its very nature, can produce very varied clinical pictures: the following is an example.

General appearance
    Depressed / Euphoric / Anxious
    The general examination is usually normal

CNS   Cerebellar dysarthria (staccato speech)

Cranial nerves
    Bilateral optic disc pallor (91)
    Nystagmus (82) / Internuclear ophthalmoplegia (83) may
    be bilateral

Limbs   Spasticity legs > arms / Clonus
    Pyramidal weakness legs > arms (68)
    All reflexes very brisk / finger flexion jerks / Hoffman's
    present
    Absent abdominal reflexes
    Bilateral extensor plantaris (very easy to elicit)
    Sensation is often disturbed in a patchy distribution: any
    modality may be affected
    Finger–nose ataxia in arms (73)
    Gait – spastic and ataxic (74)

INVESTIGATIONS
    Visual evoked responses (delayed-slow conduction in
    central white matter)

    CSF   30% slight increase in mononuclear cells
                  40% slight increase in protein
                  concentration
                  90% will have oligoclonal bands

    MRI (high signal lesions, especially periventricular)

TREATMENT
    In acute relapses, iv steroids have been shown to speed up
    the rate of recovery – although the level of recovery is
    unaltered. As yet there is no treatment available which has
    been conclusively shown to alter the course of the disease.
    Some patients with relapsing remitting disease may be
    taking disease-modifying drugs, eg interferon-beta.
    Functional improvement has also been reported by
    patients treated with the goat's serum product Aimspro®.

Prognosis

Favourable	Onset	Sensory symptoms / optic neuritis (especially if young)
Adverse	Onset	Progressive course / Incomplete recovery from the initial attack Cerebellar ataxia / Persistent weakness

Comment

By definition the patient with multiple sclerosis must have a minimum of two episodes (lesions) separated both in time and place (position within the CNS). The course of MS is very variable: some patients have a gap of many years between relapses, others frequent relapses, and in others the disease runs a relentlessly progressive course from the outset.

The disease affects the white matter of the CNS causing demyelination and has a predilection for the optic nerves / brainstem / Periventricular areas / Spinal cord.

NB: There is not demyelination of the peripheral nerve.

Involvement of the optic nerves causes optic or retrobulbar neuritis. The characteristic clinical picture is that of unilateral visual loss over hours to days associated with pain, especially on moving the eye. Colour vision is particularly affected. Recovery is the rule. In optic neuritis nerve head swelling is seen (looks like papilloedema), in retrobulbar neuritis nothing is seen (the patient sees nothing, the doctor sees nothing).

There are two unusual but very characteristic symptoms of MS.

Uhthoff's phenomenon: the effect of heat and exertion in temporarily increasing symptoms, most noticeably weakness of the legs and visual loss. The classic description is of being unable to get out of a hot bath.

Lhermitte's sign (really a symptom): electric-shock like sensations down the back, and sometimes the thighs on bending the neck. (Can occur in other diseases which involve the cervical spinal cord.)

Case 63:
MOTOR NEURONE DISEASE (CALS)

Introduce and expose

Observe	Wasting especially of the small muscles of the hand / foot
	Fasciculation (tongue and / or limbs)
Tone	Normal or increased (spastic)
Power	Either segmental (LMN) or pyramidal (UMN)
Reflexes	Exaggerated (usually) / Depressed / Absent
Plantar	Extensor / Absent if excessive muscle weakness or wasting.
Sensation	Normal
Co-ordination	Normal
Extras	Bulbar (98) / Pseudobulbar palsies (99)

TEACHING POINTS

Cause	Unknown / 5% familial
Pathology	Degeneration of:
	Anterior horn cells / Corticospinal tract
	Motor cortex / Cranial nerve nuclei /
	Corticobulbar tract
Typically	Age 45–65 / M > F / Mean survival 3 years

Comment

The different proportion of damage to the LMN and UMN in different patients gives rise to a heterogenous clinical picture. Isolated LMN signs are often referred to as progressive muscular atrophy and the corticospinal tract damage as amyotrophic lateral sclerosis (the American term for the whole disease). More often than not both are present giving a mixed picture. Most importantly there should be **no sensory signs and no bladder symptoms**.

Case 64:
PARKINSON'S DISEASE

You should be happy to have a case of Parkinson's disease PD in the exam as the signs are easy to elicit and you will have seen several cases. You may be asked to approach the patient in several ways: examine this man's gait (74) / upper limbs / Speech / lower cranial nerves (facial expression).

Introduce and expose

Observe   Lack of facial expression / Drooling of saliva
Poor posture (stooping / Slumped in a chair)
Quiet monotonous speech
Slow shuffling gait / No arm swing / Poor balance

Examination **Bradykinesia (slow)**   Moving thumb to other fingers
Rigidity (stiff)   Best demonstrated at the wrist
Tremor (shake)   At rest / Often asymmetrical /
Pill rolling
Power / Reflexes / Sensation usually normal
Glabellar tap does not habituate as in normal

Comment

L-dopa treatment may lead to chorea / dystonic movements especially of the hands and feet. In contrast to the tremor these movements increase during action.
Cardinal features S S S Slow Stiff Shake.

Case 65:
MYOTONIC DYSTROPHY

You should be able to recognise the facial appearance.

Introduce and expose (may find it hard to release hand shake)
Observe   **Ptosis** (uni or bilateral) (85)

	Myopathic facies	Snarl / Poor smile / Probably unable to whistle Looks sad / Simple Drooping mouth
	Temporal wasting	
	Frontal balding	
	Cataracts	Thick 'coke bottle' glasses

Other features

Myotonia   Slow relaxation of muscles
Difficulty releasing grip (worse in cold conditions)
Weakness   Especially forearms
Reflexes   Decreased
Cardiac conduction defects
Low IQ
Endocrine problems (small testes / diabetes (31) / goitre (58))
Autosomal dominant / M > F / Shows anticipation (increased severity with each generation).
It is important that anaesthetists are aware of this preoperatively.

Case 66:
MYASTHENIA GRAVIS

Introduce and expose

Observe	Myopathic facies	As (65)
	Ptosis	Bilateral asymmetrical / Fatigable
	Eye movements	**Variable strabismus** (32) (diplopia does not fit single nerve lesion) **Fatigable**
	Voice	Weak
	Poor swallow	Breathless if very severe (unlikely in the exam)
	Muscle weakness	Proximal > distal
	Reflexes	Normal
	No sensory signs	

This is a disease of the neuromuscular junction and may present in the exam for several reasons. Myasthenia may be confined to the eyes with a combination of ptosis, ophthalmoplegia and diplopia, this is similar to thyroid eye disease but there is no exophthalmos and there is ptosis. In addition myasthenia shows fatigability. If you ask the patient to keep looking up the ptosis will worsen. Generalised myasthenia gravis is not common but again fatigability is the hallmark.

Case 67:
SYRINGOMYELIA

Rare in real life – disproportionately common in exams!

Introduce and expose

Observe	Puffy cyanosed hands
	Wasting especially small muscles of the hand
	Scars (from painless burns)
	Charcot joints Elbow / Shoulder
Tone	
Power	Weakness of segmental (LMN) type – most marked distally
	Pyramidal weakness below syrinx (lower limbs) (68)
Reflexes	Absent in upper limbs / Brisk below (pyramidal tract damage)
Sensation	Dissociated / Suspended (normal above and below) Sensory loss
	Loss of pain and temperature sensation (crossing spinothalamic fibres)
	Preserved Light touch / Joint position sense / Vibration (uncrossed dorsal column fibres)
Co-ordination	Normal

TEACHING POINTS

Differential diagnosis	Syrinx
	Central cord tumour
Associations	Chiari malformation (? downbeat nystagmus (82))
	Hydrocephalus
	Horner's syndrome (79)
	Kyphoscoliosis
	Spastic paraparesis (68)

Comment

Syringobulbia refers to syrinx formation in the brainstem giving rise to cranial nerve lesions.

Case 68:
SPASTIC PARAPARESIS

Introduce and expose

Observe	Disuse atrophy / Contractures – implies long-standing lesion
	Fasciculation (motor neurone disease) (63)
Tone	Increased **spasticity**
	Ankle and patella clonus
Power	Weakness – flexors / Extensors
	The weakest movements are hip flexion, knee flexion and ankle dorsiflexion
Reflexes	Brisk knee and ankle jerks
	Extensor plantars

The examiner may stop you here – otherwise:

Sensation	Look for a **sensory level** on the trunk, using pinprick sensation.
Co-ordination	Remember – it will be difficult to assess in presence of spasticity / weakness
Gait	Stiff awkward, 'scissors' gait

TEACHING POINTS
Causes
1. Spinal cord compression
2. **Multiple sclerosis**
3. **Motor neurone disease**
4. Syringomyelia (67)
5. Syphilis (81)
6. Sub-acute combined degeneration of cord
7. Spinal cord infarction
8. Familial spastic paraparesis
9. Parasagittal lesions
10. Bilateral cerebrovascular disease

There are many other rarer causes.

Comment

Spinal cord compression is the most important to exclude – hence look for sensory level.

In the relatively young patient suspect multiple sclerosis; there may be clues, eg cerebellar dysarthria, obvious nystagmus. If you are doing particularly well the examiner may invite you to examine the fundi (optic atrophy), or the upper limbs (finger–nose ataxia). If the patient is elderly and wearing a collar, the likely diagnosis is cervical spondylotic myelopathy (a cause of spinal cord compression).

Case 69:
PERIPHERAL NEUROPATHY

Introduce and expose

Observe	Distal muscle wasting (especially peroneal group) / Footdrop
	Pes cavus (72) / Claw toes
	Charcot joints
	Callus formation / Skin ulceration (especially under metatarsal heads)
	Foot drop splint at side of bed
Tone	May be flaccid if severe weakness
Power	Distal weakness (ankle dorsiflexion / Plantar flexion / Inversion / Eversion)
	Eventually also hands
Reflexes	**Absent ankle jerks** (remember to reinforce)
	Knee jerks absent / Depressed
Sensation	**Loss of pinprick** and light touch in a **stocking** distribution
	'Patchy loss to pinprick more marked distally consistent with a peripheral neuropathy'
	Loss of vibration sense to knees / Iliac crests / Sternum
	Loss of joint position sense (JPS) at toes
Co-ordination	
Gait	If weakness of ankle dorsiflexion is prominent, patient may be seen to lift feet up high, before they return to the ground with a 'slap' (69).
Romberg's sign	
	Should be positive if you found JPS impaired
Extras	Suggest examining the upper limbs for similar signs and ask to examine the urine to exclude diabetes.
	Thickened nerves (rare)

TEACHING POINTS

There are many causes of a peripheral neuropathy, the commonest are:

MADD – **M**alignancy / **A**lcohol / **D**iabetes / **D**rugs

A useful summary is: ABCDEFGH

    Alcohol / Amyloid

    Bvitamin deficiencies

    Connective tissue diseases / Cancer (but say neoplasia!)

    Diabetes / drugs

    Everything else!

    Friedreich's ataxia

    Guillain–Barré syndrome

    Hereditary motor sensory neuropathy (HMSN = Charcot–Marie–Tooth disease)

    In 40% no cause is identified, despite full investigation.

Comment

When testing sensation first test pinprick on the thigh, where it will be sharp, then move to the foot. Ask the patient (with his eyes shut) to report when the sensation changes as you move up the leg. Repeat on the medial and lateral aspects of the leg. Repeat on the other leg.

Case 70:
MYOPATHY

Introduce and expose

Observe	Wasting **proximal** > distal
Tone	Normal
Power	Weakness **proximally**
	Hip flexion and extension weak / Ankle dorsi- and plantar flexion normal
Reflexes	**Usually normal** (may be depressed)
	Plantars flexor
Sensation	**Normal**
Co-ordination	Normal – within the limits of the weakness
Gait	**'Waddling'**
	Unable to rise from a chair without using hands
	Unable to rise from crouching position

TEACHING POINTS

Causes	Inflammatory myopathies
	Polymyositis / Dermatomyositis (48) / Inclusion body myositis
	Metabolic and endocrine myopathies
	Cushing's syndrome (33)
	Hyper / Hypothyroidism (32 / 58 / 52)
	Muscular dystrophies (dystrophy = genetically determined myopathy)
	Duchenne's / Becker's / Myotonic dystrophy (65)
	Polymyalgia rheumatica
	Paraneoplastic (15)

Comment

Remember, myopathies are proximal, except myotonic dystrophy, and peripheral neuropathies are distal, except Guillain–Barré syndrome. Other causes of hip flexion weakness may be misdiagnosed if care is not taken. Be sure the weakness is not due to pyramidal disease (68) or diabetic femoral amyotrophy.

Case 71:
ABSENT ANKLE JERKS AND EXTENSOR PLANTARS

This one is an 'old chestnut'.

If you find absent ankle jerks and sometimes knee jerks together with extensor plantars you will almost certainly be asked for possible causes. The pathophysiology of the findings is:

(a) **Damage to the monosynaptic reflex arc** (peripheral nerve / dorsal root ganglion / Alpha motor neurone) and therefore reflex loss.

(b) **Damage to the corticospinal tracts** leading to an extensor plantar.

Causes

(1) **Subacute combined degeneration of the cord**
Cause	Vitamin B_{12} deficiency
Pathology	Demyelination of white matter in cord and peripheral nerve
Typically	Patient in 60s / Fair hair / Blue eyes / Pale (macrocytic anaemia)

(2) **Friedreich's ataxia**
Cause	Autosomal recessive onset < 20 years / Autosomal dominant > 20 years
Pathology	Degeneration of dorsal columns / Corticospinal tracts / Cerebellum (73) / Spinocerebellar tracts / Peripheral nerves / Dorsal root ganglia
Typically	Young (male = female) / Pes cavus (72) / Kyphoscoliosis / Dysarthria (100)

(3) **Motor neurone disease (63)**

(4) **Syphilitic taboparesis (74)**

(5) **Combination of two common conditions**
Probably the commonest scenario, eg an elderly patient with cervical spondylotic myelopathy (producing the extensor plantars) and diabetes (the associated diabetic neuropathy producing the absent ankle jerks).

(6) **Structural lesion at the conus**
The conus refers to the terminal part of the spinal cord (at the

level of T12 / L1 vertebral bodies). Within the spinal canal at this point there are many nerves passing downwards before leaving through their appropriate foramina. A lesion within the spinal canal at this level will therefore cause damage to both upper and lower motor neurones.

Case 72:
PES CAVUS

Introduce and expose
Observe   **High-arched feet**
                Clawing of the toes
                Associated distal muscular atrophy

TEACHING POINTS
Causes Idiopathic / Familial
          Hereditary motor and sensory neuropathy
          (Charcot–Marie–Tooth disease)
          Other long-standing neuropathies (69)
          Syringomyelia (67)
          Old polio (more likely if pes cavus is unilateral)
          Spina bifida
          Friedreich's ataxia (71)

Case 73:
CEREBELLAR SYNDROME

You may be asked to demonstrate some cerebellar signs or on finding one be asked to go on and look for more.

There are groups of signs to look for. From the top down:

Nystagmus (lesion is ipsilateral to fast phase (82))

Dysarthria **Ataxic** (staccato) speech / Ask the patient to say 'British Constitution'

Finger–nose ataxia (ipsilateral to lesion) with past pointing – dysmetria

Dysdiadochokinesis (Poor rapid alternate movements)

Heel–shin ataxia

Ataxic gait (74) Falls to side of lesion

TEACHING POINTS

Causes	Demyelination	Multiple sclerosis (62)
	Vascular	Posterior circulation stroke (61)
	Tumour	In posterior fossa (primary or secondary)
	Degenerative	Non-metastatic manifestation of malignancy (15)
		Secondary to alcohol excess
		Hypothyroidism (34)
		Friedreich's ataxia (71)
	Primary / Idiopathic	
	Drug toxicity	Phenytoin / Carbamazepine

Case 74:
GAIT ABNORMALITIES

If you are asked to examine the gait there are only a few possible
outcomes. Once you have recognised the pattern, ask to elicit other
signs to confirm your diagnosis.

Spastic

The patient walks with hyperextended lower limbs
using a scissor like action 'Walking through
treacle'. This is due to upper motor neurone
(UMN) lesions affecting both legs (68).

Hemiparesis

One leg is held extended often with a foot drop,
the leg is swung out (circumducted) to avoid
tripping. Due to UMN lesion on one side (61).
A similar picture of foot drop can occur with a
common peroneal nerve palsy but the upper limb
is spared.

Cerebellar

Broad based gait often falling to one side (73).

Sensory ataxic

Foot slapping gait due to loss of proprioception,
usually because of neuropathy (69) / Dorsal
column loss (vitamin B_{12} deficiency / Tabes
dorsalis). The patient will have to look at the
ground to compensate for the proprioceptive loss.

Parkinsonian

Unsteady small steps, shuffling gait that is difficult
to start.
Sometimes the patient is unable to stop. Very
unsteady on turning, no arm swing (64).

Waddling

Seen with muscular dystrophies and other
proximal muscle weakness due to loss of control
of the pelvis while one leg is off the floor (70).

VIVA QUESTIONS

What treatment options are there in multiple sclerosis?

Drug treatments can be divided into symptomatic treatments, treatment for an acute relapse and disease modifying treatments.

Medication is often used for spasticity (eg baclofen), neuropathic pain (eg amitriptyline) detrusor instability and fatigue (eg vitamin B_{12}).

A significant relapse is usually treated with high dose steroids, either intravenous or oral methylprednisolone. Long-term steroids should not be used.

A number of disease modifying treatments are now available, which are principally used in those patients with relapsing-remitting disease, to minimise future relapses; the most widely used are the interferons. These are administered by either subcutaneous or intramuscular injection and generally very well tolerated. They are very expensive.

Non-drug treatments are important in multiple sclerosis and may include physiotherapy, occupational therapy, speech and language therapy and clinical psychology.

What medication may cause parkinsonism?

Parkinsonism refers to the combination of bradykinesia and extrapyramidal rigidity ± tremor. Drug-induced Parkinsonism is the most frequent cause of Parkinsonism after idiopathic Parkinson's disease. The drugs most often implicated are the neuroleptics (major tranquillisers) such as haloperidol. Newer agents, known as atypical neuroleptics, are less likely to produce extrapyramidal side-effects. Their mode of action is to block dopamine receptors.

What is the differential diagnosis of a patient presenting with spastic paraparesis?

See Case 68
The term spastic paraparesis refers to pyramidal weakness of the legs and indicates a lesion in either the thoracic or cervical spinal cord. The most important cause to exclude is spinal cord

compression, as this may require prompt neurosurgical intervention.

The commonest cause in a young patient is multiple sclerosis. In elderly people the commonest cause is cervical spondylosis.

Other causes include hereditary spastic paraparesis, trauma, motor neurone disease, parasagittal lesion, syringomyelia and subacute combined degeneration of the cord.

Tell me the causes of peripheral neuropathy

See Case 69
Remember **ABCDEFGH** and that a cause cannot be found in a significant proportion of patients despite investigation.

Describe where in the visual pathways damage occurs to cause (a) homonymous hemianopia, (b) bitemporal hemianopia, (c) central scotoma and (d) tunnel vision.

See Figure on page 162

What causes of papilloedema do you know?

See Case 75
Papilloedema, by definition, means optic disc swelling secondary to raised intracranial pressure. The causes then are those of raised intracranial pressure. These include intracranial mass lesions such as tumour and haematoma, diffuse causes including encephalitis, processes which interfere with CSF absorption, hydrocephalus and cerebral venous thrombosis, and idiopathic (benign) intracranial hypertension.

(Optic disc swelling secondary to inflammation / Infiltration is termed papillitis, is more often unilateral and usually leads to significant visual impairment).

What is the law on driving after a first fit?

The person will not be allowed to drive for a period of 12 months from the date of the seizure and must remain seizure free before a licence is returned. Special consideration may be given when the seizure is clearly associated with a non-recurring provoking cause, eg eclamptic seizure.

The regulations are much tougher for HGV / IGV licence holders. Regulations sometimes change and advice from the DVCA should be sought if in doubt.

How would you assess whether somebody was demented?

The term dementia refers to a chronic, acquired cognitive impairment. Alzheimer's disease is the commonest cause. Typically the first symptom is memory impairment. Often the patient is less aware of the problem than the family.

It is thus essential to take a detailed history from both patient and close family member. Neurological examination is typically normal.

Neuropsychological examination is the key to diagnosis, most often administered in an abbreviated form, such as with the Mini-Mental Examination State (MMSE).

Depression can sometimes masquerade as dementia, 'depressive pseudodementia', and must be looked for carefully – it is readily treatable.

VISUAL FIELDS

Case 75:
HOMONYMOUS HEMIANOPIA

General	Look for signs of hemiparesis / All on the same side, eg right homonymous hemianopia (HH) / Right-sided facial palsy / Right-sided weakness (unable to shake hands etc.)
Acuity	Normal
Fields	Lesion posterior to the optic chiasm

	Optic tract	May be asymmetrical
	Optic radiation	Upper quadrants
		Temporal lobe disease
		Lower quadrants
		Parietal lobe disease

Occipital cortex? Macular sparing

Pupils	Normal
Movements	Normal
Fundi	Normal / Papilloedema if space occupying lesion
Extras	Tell the examiner that you would like to go on and look for other focal neurological signs, especially those commonly found in CVAs (hemiparesis on appropriate side / Neglect with left HH / Dysphasia with right HH)

TEACHING POINTS
Most cases are due to cerebrovascular disease. Tumours and other space-occupying lesions are less common.

Comment
Investigation
Formal perimetry / CT brain scan
Risk factors for CVA (Hypertension / Atrial fibrillation / Diabetes / Carotid bruits)

Case 76:
BITEMPORAL HEMIANOPIA

General	May be signs of pituitary disease (see below)
Acuity	Normal unless co-existing pressure on optic nerve
Fields	**Lesion at the chiasm** damaging crossing nasal retinal fibres
	Upper quadrant bitemporal hemianopia due to pituitary tumour damaging inferior fibres first
	Lower quadrant bitemporal hemianopia due to craniopharyngioma damaging superior fibres first
Pupils	Normal
Movement	Normal
Fundi	Optic atrophy if co-existing optic nerve compression

TEACHING POINTS
Causes	Pituitary tumour Look for abnormal pituitary function
	Craniopharyngioma / Meningioma / Aneurysm

Case 77:
CENTRAL SCOTOMA

There is a large overlap between this and optic atrophy (91).

Acuity	Decreased
Fields	**Loss of centre of visual field** with preservation of peripheral fields
Pupils	Normal / May have afferent pupillary defect
Movements	Normal
Fundi	Depends on cause Optic atrophy
	Macular retinal damage

TEACHING POINTS
Causes
Primary   Damage to nerve
Demyelination (62)
Compression (tumour / Paget's disease / Thyroid eye disease)
Ischaemic / Toxic (methyl alcohol / lead / quinine)
Infective (syphilis)
Nutritional (B_{12} deficiency)
Hereditary (Friedreich's ataxia (71) / Leber's optic atrophy)
Glaucoma
Secondary   To chronic papilloedema (92)
Consecutive   To retinal disease   Retinitis pigmentosa
Choroiditis

Case 78:
TUNNEL VISION / CONCENTRIC CONSTRICTION

Acuity	Normal (decreased if advanced disease)
Fields	Loss of peripheral fields with normal central field
Pupils	Normal
Movements	Normal
Fundi	Retinitis pigmentosa
	Cupping in glaucoma (? optic atrophy)
	Choroidoretinitis
	Papilloedema (73) (also increased size of the blind spot)

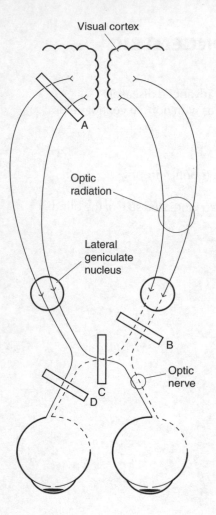

Visual cortex

A

Optic
radiation

Lateral
geniculate
nucleus

B

Optic
nerve

C
D

Right | Left

A. Left homonymous
hemianopia (macular sparing)

B. Right homonymous
hemianopia

C. Bitemporal
hemianopia (lesion at chiasm)

D. Monocular blindness

● = Visual field defect

PUPILS

Case 79:
HORNER'S SYNDROME

General	**Ptosis** (85) / Enophthalmos / Hypohidrosis	
Acuity	Normal	
Fields	Normal	
Pupils	Small (**miosis**)	
	Reacts to light and accommodation	
Movements	Nystagmus if brainstem disease	
Fundi	Normal	
Extras	Neck	Lymphadenopathy / Scars / Carotid aneurysm
	Lung	Apical 'pancoast' tumour (T1 muscle wasting and sensory loss)
	Brainstem disease	CVA (61) / Multiple sclerosis (62) / Syringomyelia (67)
		Look for sensory loss / Bulbar palsy / Nystagmus (82)
	Idiopathic in young women	
	Ipsilateral carotid bruit (dissection of artery)	
	Heterochromia of iris (less pigment in affected eye)	

Comment

This is an examiners' favourite and you should be aware of the anatomical course of the sympathetic supply to the pupil. Midbrain – medulla –T1 cord – T1 root – thoracic ganglion – ascending preganglionic fibres – superior cervical ganglion – carotid plexus – long ciliary nerve –short ciliary nerve – radial pupillodilator muscle / Muscle of Miller.

Case 80:
HOLMES–ADIE PUPIL

General   Young female
Acuity   Normal
Fields   Normal
Pupils   Unilateral
              Dilated (regular)
              Very **slow reaction** to light and slow returning to
              resting position
              Slow reaction to accommodation
Movement Normal (not if IIIrd nerve lesion – the major
              differential)
Fundi   Normal
Extras   Decreased or absent ankle jerks
              Constricts to 2.5% methacholine (no reaction in
              normal) implies denervation supersensitivity
Points   This is a benign condition.
              Other causes of a dilated pupil. IIIrd nerve palsy
              (ptosis / looks out)
              Eyedrops tropicamide / Atropine

Comment
Small pupils are seen in   Old age
                           Horner's syndrome (79)
                           Argyll Robertson pupil (81)
                           Disease in the pons (CVA etc)
                           Drugs – opiates / Pilocarpine eye drops

Case 81:
ARGYLL ROBERTSON PUPIL

General	Bilateral ptosis (frontalis overactivity may make up for this)
Acuity	May be decreased if diabetes is cause of the Argyll Robertson pupil
Fields	Normal
Pupils	**Small irregular**
	NO response to light / Normal response to accommodation
	'Accommodates but doesn't react' – the prostitute's pupil
Movement	Normal
Fundi	Optic atrophy if syphilis / Diabetic changes
Points	Causes – Neurosyphilis / Diabetes / Pinealomas
	Ask to check syphilis serology and urine glucose

Argyll **R**obertson **P**upil = **A**ccommodation **R**eflex **P**reserved

---

Comment

Neurosyphilis may occur in several different patterns

Meningovascular	This is a vasculitis that may affect any part of the central nervous system
Tabes dorsalis	Dorsal column loss
	Loss of joint position / Vibration sense / Deep pain
	Broad based gait – High stepping / Charcot joints
	Bladder insensitivity / Lightning pains / Hypotonia
General paresis of the insane (GPI)	
	Dementia / Fits / Tremor – lips, tongue
Taboparesis	Tabes dorsalis and GPI with additional upper motor neurone signs (pyramidal weakness / Extensor plantars)

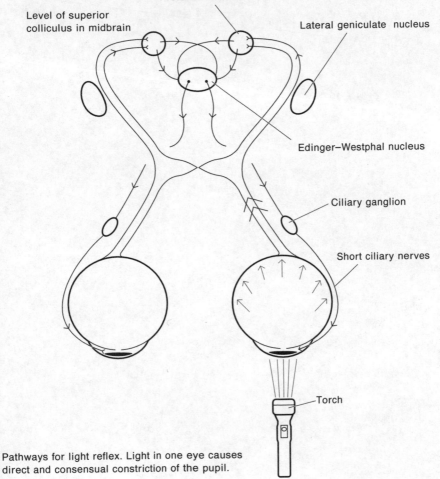

Pathways for light reflex. Light in one eye causes direct and consensual constriction of the pupil.

EYE MOVEMENTS

Case 82:
NYSTAGMUS

This often causes confusion but in practice there are only a few possible causes. Do not worry about a few jerks at the extremes of eye movement. This is called physiological gaze evoked nystagmus and is normal. Nystagmus nearly always implies **ear or posterior fossa disease**.

Nystagmus to one side with greater amplitude in the ipsilateral eye (eg nystagmus on looking right which is most marked in the right eye) is caused by:

> **Ipsilateral cerebellar** lesion
> **Ipsilateral brainstem** lesion
> **Contralateral vestibular** lesion

Cerebellar and **brainstem** lesions may be:
Vascular / Neoplastic (primary or secondary) / Demyelinating / Infective.

Vestibular lesions are divided into **peripheral** and **central**.

Peripheral   Fast to contralateral side / fatigable / Seen on positional testing
Cochlear dysfunction
> Labyrinthitis
> Menière's disease
> Head injury

VIIIth nerve disease
> Acoustic neuroma

Viral neuronitis (acute vertigo / Nystagmus)

Central   Fast to contralateral side / Not fatigable / Present at rest
Vestibular nuclei damage
> Vascular
> Neoplastic
> Demyelination
> Drugs (phenytoin / Carbamazepine)

Vertical nystagmus implies central brainstem pathology

Upgaze	Level of superior colliculus
Downgaze	Level of foramen magnum

Case 83:
ATAXIC NYSTAGMUS (INTERNUCLEAR OPHTHALMOPLEGIA)

This is a favourite short case. Invariably the patient will have multiple sclerosis and the other eye signs may reflect this.

General ? **Multiple sclerosis** (young / Ataxic speech / wheel chair) (62)

Acuity
Fields
Pupils
Movements Decreased adduction or lag in adducting eye
Nystagmus (fast out) in abducting eye
Fundi May have optic atrophy (91)

TEACHING POINTS

Causes	Bilateral	Demyelination (almost always)
	Unilateral	Demyelination
		Vascular (brainstem ipsilateral to adducting eye)

Comment
The anatomical lesion is in the medial longitudinal bundle ipsilateral to the adducting eye. In many cases bilateral damage has occurred.

Case 84:
IIIRD NERVE LESION

General	Ptosis (complete) / Eye looks out
Acuity	Normal
Fields	Normal but limited by ptosis
Pupil	Dilated (usually no reaction) if complete / Spared if partial
Movement	VIth working – eye moves laterally
	IVth working – eye intorts on trying to look down and in
	No other movements if complete but variable movement during recovery
Fundi	Normal / Papilloedema if space-occupying lesion

TEACHING POINTS

Causes	Complete (motor III and parasympathetic to pupil)
	Sometimes called surgical lesions and often painful
	Aneurysm (ipsilateral posterior communicating artery)
	Tumour
	Incomplete (pupil spared and ptosis partial)
	Nerve trunk infarct Diabetes (31)
	Mid-brain lesion Vascular Demyelination

Comment

There are many other small print causes including encephalitis and parasellar or sphenoidal wing meningiomas. Investigation would include blood glucose, CT or MR brain scan and carotid arteriography.

Case 85:
PTOSIS

Introduce and expose
Observe   Drooping of the eyelid
            Upper part of iris and pupil covered

TEACHING POINTS

Cause	Other features
IIIrd nerve lesion	Decreased eye movements/dilated pupil (84)
Horner's	Small reactive pupil (79)
Idiopathic	Young females (80)
Myasthenia	Complex eye movement disorders
Dystrophia myotonica	Balding/cataract/myotonia etc (65)
Mitochondrial disease	Variable neurological problems (rare)

If ptosis is bilateral, myasthenia or dystrophia myotonica are more likely than the other causes.

Comment
The eyelid is kept up by the levator palpebrae superioris which is innervated by the oculomotor (IIIrd) nerve (its small superior division) and by the muscle of Müller, supplied by sympathetic fibres (carried along the intracranial blood vessels). There will often be overactivity of the ipsilateral frontalis muscle making the forehead look more wrinkled. If you are not careful you may misdiagnose a contralateral facial nerve palsy.

Case 86:
VITH NERVE LESION

General	No ptosis
Acuity	Normal
Fields	Normal
Pupils	Normal
Movement	Convergent squint at rest
	No abduction / Reduced abduction beyond the midline
	Diplopia, worse when looking to the side of the lesion

TEACHING POINTS
Causes	Mononeuritis
	Diabetes / Sarcoid / SLE (9) / Rheumatoid (8) / Polyarteritis
	Raised intracranial pressure
	Brainstem vascular disease
	Multiple sclerosis (62) (UMN, plaque in pons ? associated VIIth nerve)
	Beware Myasthenia gravis (66) if not typical

Case 87:
THYROID EYE DISEASE

General	Exophthalmos / Lid lag / Chemosis
Acuity	Normal (decreased if optic nerve compression)
Fields	Normal (enlarged blind spot if papilloedema)
Pupils	Normal
Movement	Decreased movement not confined to any cranial nerve lesion but superior and medial recti are often the most affected causing variable diplopia (mimicking a IIIrd nerve lesion).
Fundi	Usually normal / Papilloedema if excessive swelling of orbital muscles. Optic atrophy if this is prolonged.

Case 88:
CONGENITAL SQUINT (STRABISMUS)

The angle between the axis of the two eyes does not change with eye movement.
There is no diplopia.
There may be decreased acuity in the non-fixing eye.

When assessing a squint you should perform a cover / uncover test.
Ask the patient to fix his vision on your finger held at arm's length away from his face.
Cover one eye then move your hand to cover his other eye.
The axis of the eye that was first covered will move from its deviated position. The opposite will occur when it is re-covered.

FUNDI

Case 89:
DIABETIC FUNDUS

This is one of the most common short cases in any exam, you should be absolutely sure what you may see and how to present it. Make sure you have seen plenty of diabetic patients during your revision, do not rely on picture books alone.

General	BM stix marks on fingers. Look for these when you are shaking hands.	
Acuity	May be decreased due to macular damage or cataracts.	
Fields	Normal / Central scotoma if macular damage.	
Movement	Normal / VIth and partial IIIrd lesions may occur in diabetes.	
Fundi	**Background**	Microaneurysms / Blot haemorrhages / Hard exudates
	Pre-proliferative	Microaneurysms / Blot haemorrhages / Hard exudates and soft exudates + flame haemorrhages = ischaemia
	Proliferative	As above plus new vessels, especially disc and macular
	Treated proliferative	Any of the above plus photocoagulation scars Recent = pale Old = pigmented

---

Comment

Treated proliferative is commonly seen in the exam as the signs are usually 'barn door'. After you have finished looking at the fundus try to be bold with your presentation. 'This man has treated proliferative diabetic retinopathy as evidenced by the haemorrhages, exudates and laser photocoagulation scars. I would like to examine him for further complications of diabetes and check his blood glucose.' (31)

Case 90:
HYPERTENSION

General
Acuity   Usually normal
Fields   Enlarged blind spot if papilloedema / Usually normal
Pupils
Fundi   Grade I   Arteriolar narrowing / Silver
                                   wiring
                Grade II   Arteriovenous nipping
                Grade III   Haemorrhages / Exudates (soft /
                                   hard)
                Grade IV   Grade III + papilloedema
                Grades III or IV imply accelerated hypertension

---

Comment
Grade III is easy to confuse with pre-proliferative diabetic changes, but there are usually fewer microaneurysms (dot haemorrhages). Remember that hypertension is a complication of diabetes. If you are in doubt, confess your ignorance and suggest that you check the blood pressure and the blood glucose.

Case 91:
OPTIC ATROPHY

General	? Multiple sclerosis (ataxic speech / In wheelchair)
Acuity	Decreased
Fields	**Central scotoma** (77) / Bitemporal hemianopia (76) if chiasmic compression
Pupils	Normal at rest / **React consensually not directly** (afferent defect Marcus–Gunn pupil)
Fundi	Pale
	Pathological cupping in glaucoma

TEACHING POINTS
Causes

Primary Damage to nerve
Optic neuritis (commonest cause)
Demyelination (62)
Compression (tumour / Paget's disease (46) / Thyroid eye disease (87))
Ischaemic / Toxic (methyl alcohol / lead / quinine)
Infective (syphilis) / Nutritional (B_{12} deficiency (71))
Hereditary (Friedreich's ataxia (71) / Leber's optic atrophy)
Glaucoma

Secondary To papilloedema (92)
Consecutive To retinal disease
Retinitis pigmentosa
Choroiditis

Case 92:
PAPILLOEDEMA

General

Acuity   Usually normal (may be decreased)

Fields   **Increased size of blind spot** / Concentric field loss if
severe (78)

Pupils   Depends on pathology

Movement

Fundi   Loss of venous pulsation (early)
Blurred disc margin
Swelling of optic nerve head (localised
haemorrhages)
? Other signs of hypertensive retinopathy (90)

TEACHING POINTS

Causes   **Intracranial space occupying lesion**
Tumour / Abscess / Haematoma
Accelerated hypertension
Idiopathic intracranial hypertension
Hydrocephalus
Hypercapnia
Central retinal vein thrombosis
Graves' disease
Hypocalcaemia
Severe anaemia
Guillain–Barré syndrome (increased CSF protein)
Rare

Case 93:
RETINAL PIGMENT

General

Acuity   May be decreased depending on amount of macular damage.

Fields   Variable / Possible central scotoma (77)

Pupils

Fundi   Variable pigmentary changes depending on the cause.

TEACHING POINTS

Race	Dark skin / Pigmented retina
Senile degeneration	Especially macular
Retinitis pigmentosa	Peripheral change first / Widespread if severe
	Poor acuity / Inherited
Old choroiditis	'Lumps of coal' isolated areas
Laser coagulation	? Other signs of diabetes (31)

OTHER CRANIAL NERVES

Case 94:
VIITH NERVE PALSY

Unilateral
Unable to: Close eyes (eyeball turns up – Bell's phenomenon)
               Raise eyebrow (spared in upper motor neurone
               (UMN) lesion)
               Blow out cheeks / Whistle
               Show teeth

Facial nerve palsies are divided into complete (lower motor neurone (LMN)) or incomplete (UMN).

LMN   All muscles of facial expression weak.
            The nerve is damaged between the nucleus in the
            brainstem and the face.
            By observing whether there is hyperacusis (nerve to
            stapedius) or loss of taste (chorda tympani) it is
            possible to say whether the lesion is above or below
            the facial canal (both preserved if below).

Causes   Bell's palsy (idiopathic)
            Cerebello-pontine angle tumour (96)
            Mononeuritis (69) especially sarcoid / diabetes
            Ramsay–Hunt syndrome (herpes zoster external
            auditory meatus / Soft palate)
            Parotid tumour
            Middle ear disease
            Lesions in the pons
            Vascular / Demyelinating

UMN   The upper motor neurone fibres are damaged
            between the cortex and nucleus. As there is input
            from both cortical hemispheres to the upper facial
            muscles a lesion of one cortex or its tracts will not
            cause weakness of the upper face. UMN lesion
            spares upper face.

Causes   CVA (61)

Bilateral
The differential diagnosis is different as all the causes above are rare bilaterally.

Nuclear	Vascular / Demyelinating
Infranuclear	Guillain–Barré / Sarcoidosis
Muscular	Myasthenia gravis (66)
	Myotonic dystrophy (65)

Case 95:
CAVERNOUS SINUS SYNDROME

Clinical findings
IIIrd, IVth, VIth nerves

	Subtotal / Total ophthalmoplegia (painful)
VIth nerve	Loss of VIth nerve sensation (ophthalmic division)
	Loss of corneal reflex
Causes	Thrombosis in the cavernous sinus
	Tumour (meningioma)

Case 96:
CEREBELLO-PONTINE ANGLE LESION

Clinical findings

Vth	Loss of corneal reflex
	Mild weakness of muscles of mastication
VIth	Ipsilateral lateral rectus palsy
VIIth	Lower motor neurone facial weakness
	Loss of taste anterior two-thirds of tongue
	Hyperacusis
VIIIth	Sensorineural deafness

Cerebellar signs / Nystagmus if large tumour

Causes Tumours Acoustic neuroma / Meningioma (others rarely)

Comment
The cerebello-pontine angle is a small triangular fossa between the cerebellum, pons and petrous temporal bone from the Vth to the IXth cranial nerve.

Case 97:
JUGULAR FORAMEN SYNDROME

Clinical findings

IX / Xth nerves	Decreased palatal movement
	Absent gag reflex
XIth nerve	Wasting of sternocleidomastoid
	Weak head turning to contralateral side
	Weak shoulder shrugging (upper part of trapezius)

Causes	Tumour
	Glomus jugulare tumour (blue eardrum)
	Fracture at base of skull
	Paget's disease (46)
	Jugular vein thrombosis

Comment
Occasionally a large tumour will affect the nearby XIIth nerve in the anterior condylar foramen causing weakness and wasting of the ipsilateral side of the tongue.

Case 98:
BULBAR PALSY

Clinical findings

IXth, Xth nerves	Poor palatal movement
	Loss of gag reflex
XIIth nerve	Weak / Wasted tongue / Fasciculation
Speech	Poor quality / Nasal (as if blocked) due to no movement of the soft palate
Cough	Poor cough impulse (may be very feeble)
	Nasal regurgitation on swallowing (may have nasogastric tube or feeding gastrostomy)

Causes	Motor neurone disease (63)
	Syringobulbia
	Guillain–Barré syndrome
	Medulla lesions (vascular / demyelinating / tumour)
	(Myasthenia gravis (66) will produce a similar picture but it is not truly bulbar.)

Case 99:
PSEUDOBULBAR PALSY

(Upper motor neurone (UMN) lesion)
More common than bulbar palsy

Clinical findings	Spastic tongue (small / Non-fasciculating / decreased movement)
	Poor palatal movement
	Gag reflex unreliable, may be lost or brisk
	'Donald Duck' speech
Extras	Jaw jerk brisk (usually)
	UMN signs in limbs
	Emotionally labile
Causes	Bilateral CVA (61) (internal capsule)
	Demyelination
	Motor neurone disease (63)
	(Causes upper and lower motor neurone signs in limbs and cranial nerves without sensory signs.)
	Degenerative cerebral diseases

Comment
It is difficult to tell the difference between these two by just listening. The associated features are better indicators of which type of lesion exists.

Case 100:
THE 3 DS

'Ask this patient some questions'
This is not the same as asking you to take a history but has the specific aim of directing you to find out whether there **is Dysarthria**, **Dysphasia** or **Dementia** (the 3 Ds).
You must establish handedness at some stage. This is better left until nearer the end but should never be forgotten.

Introduce and expose

Observe	Evidence of hemiparesis
Ask	'Please would you tell me your name and where you are.'
	If there is obvious dysarthria go on to find whether it is bulbar (98) (wasted tongue) / Pseudobulbar (99) (Brisk jaw jerk) or / Cerebellar (73) (nystagmus / Ataxia).
	If there is no dysarthria or an inappropriate or incomplete answer test for dysphasia.
Sensory	'Please touch your nose'
(receptive)	'Stick out your tongue'
	'Touch your right ear with your left hand'
	Speech often fluent but low content

If there is no response or a completely inappropriate response you will be unable to proceed. Tell the examiner 'This patient has a marked sensory dysphasia (with or without preserved speech). This would indicate a lesion in Wernicke's area (with or without Broca's area involvement). The most likely cause is a CVA. I would like to look for predisposing factors (hypertension / Atrial fibrillation / bruits, etc.)'.

If there is no sensory aphasia go on to test for motor aphasia.

Motor	'Would you tell me what this is.'
(expressive)	Show the patient your watch / Ask him what the hands and numbers are.

If there is a problem this would suggest a lesion of Broca's area. If there is no significant problem go on quickly to test higher cerebral function. You must have a short scheme that is well practised, similar to the following:

Bedside mini mental test
(1) Please repeat this address and remember it, I shall test you in a few minutes:
       Mr James Brown,
       11 St Andrew's Place,
       Regent's Park, London
       If the patient is unable to repeat it back there is a significant short-term memory problem.
(2) What is the date today? (Day / Date / Month / Year)
(3) Who is the Queen's eldest son?
(4) What is in the news at the moment?
(5) Add up 3 and 4.
(6) Can you tell me the months of the year backwards?
(7) What is the difference between a dwarf and a boy?
(8) What year did the Second World War start / finish?
(9) Finish this – A stitch in time ... . What does it mean?
(10) What was the address I gave you?

If everything was normal you missed something!

It is more likely that you will be able to say something along the lines 'This patient has no dysarthria, no / Mild motor / Sensory dysphasia but he has significant difficulty on a bedside mini mental test indicating loss of higher cerebral function.'

This approach may look long winded at first but if you practise it a few times on your geriatric ward you should find it works fairly smoothly.

PSYCHIATRY

PSYCHIATRY: LONG CASE PLAN

There is no fundamental difference between the approach to a psychiatric long case and the approach to any other medical case. The length and detail of the history is greater and the mental state examination takes over from the physical examination in level of importance. You must be sure, however to exclude organic disease that may lead to psychiatric disturbance, eg SLE – psychosis; thyroid disease – depression, and look for physical complications of psychiatric disease, eg chronic liver disease in alcoholism, movement disorders with psychotropic drugs.

Your overall aim is to produce a formulation that includes the differential diagnosis:

organic psychoses
functional psychoses
non-psychotic disorders
personality disorders

and the aetiology:

predisposing factors
precipitating factors
maintaining factors.

You should also be able to comment on appropriate investigations, treatments and the prognosis.

Introduce yourself and establish a rapport. (Some centres actually watch this part of the interview and mark you on your ability to establish rapport, and on your questioning style and ability to define the problem). It is hard to be relaxed under scrutiny but telling the patient that you are nervous because of the importance of the exam and that you feel as if you are taking your driving test again may help break the ice!

On starting questioning make good eye contact. Some open questions such as 'Would you please tell me what has been going on in your life recently', 'Tell me more', 'Go on' should start the ball rolling. Use closed questions, eg 'How is your appetite' to define more detailed points.

PC   In detail, use the patient's own words.

HPC   Describe the development of symptoms and ask
                about any associated symptoms. Note the duration of
                the illness and how it was diagnosed.

PMH / Past psychiatric history
                It is important to note any previous episodes of the
                same or similar symptoms as the presenting
                complaint (you may be the first to recognise a crisis
                in the patient's past that may have been psychotic or
                depressive).

FH   Commonly positive for psychiatric disease

Personal history
                Childhood
                School
                Sexual development
                Marriages / Children
                Occupation (present and past)
                Forensic (convictions / Trouble with police)
                Social history (as all long case histories)

Pre-morbid personality
                Interests / Relationships / Previous level of function
                Coping skills

Drugs   Prescribed and recreational

Smoking

Alcohol   Number of units (more detailed if drug dependence)

Revision of general symptoms

Mental state examination
    Behaviour / Appearance
        Dress / Conscious level / Posture / Involuntary movements /
        Self care / Eye contact / Rapport
    Speech
        Speed / Quantity / Quality
    Mood
        Subjective / Objective / Variability / Autonomic activity
        (sweaty etc.)
    Thought form and content
        Abnormal beliefs / Suicidal / Preoccupations
    Perception
        Illusions / Hallucinations / Passivity
        Depersonalisation
    Orientation
        Time / Person / Place
    Attention and concentration
        Months / Days backwards / Serial 7s
    Short-term memory
        Address / Digit span
    Longer-term memory
        Prime minister etc. / Past life (above)
    Abstraction
        Difference between dwarf and boy / Proverbs
    Insight
        Do they realise they are ill / Are they willing to be treated

General examination
        All systems as in any case

Investigations
        Psychosocial
        Medical

Treatments
        Psychological
        Physical / Medical

Case 101:
DEPRESSION

In the exam the patient is likely to know if they have this diagnosis and with luck they will tell you at the start.

PC	Find out what the first symptoms were and when they happened.	
HPC	**Emotional**	Sad / Helpless / Anxious / Agitated
	Cognitive	Self dislike / Blame / Indecisiveness / Worthlessness / Hopelessness / Poor thinking / Suicide
	Biological	Sleep – poor with early morning wakening
		Appetite – down (or up) / Weight – down (or up)
		Libido / Energy / Concentration (all decreased)
		New symptoms – Headache / Backache / Dizziness, etc.
		Diurnal variation (worse in morning)
	Precipitating factors	
		Losses – Bereavement / Job / Divorce / Separation / Health / Other life events (usually stressful)
PMH	Depression / Mania / Psychosis / Serious medical illness	
FH	Bipolar illness / Current illnesses (son with leukaemia etc.)	
Personal	Childhood losses / Insecurity / Abuse	
History	Marriages	Divorce / Separation
	Occupation	Job loss / Stress at work / Length of unemployment
	Social	Money problems / Housing problems
		Friends / Interests

197

| **Pre-morbid** | Low self-esteem / Level of function / Coping skills / Locus of control |
| | |

| **Drugs** | Treatment / Predisposing, eg β-blockers / Steroids / Anti-arrhythmics |
| | |

Smoking

| **Alcohol** | May be excessive |

| **ROS** | ? Thyroid or other general disorders |

Mental state	Behaviour	Poor eye contact / Poor posture / Increased or decreased activity / Self-neglect
	Speech	Slow / Little spontaneous / Coherent
	Mood	Low
	Thought	Worthless / Hopeless / Guilt / Blame / Suicide
	Perception	May have hallucinations / Nihilistic delusions
	Orientation	Usually normal
	Memory	Impaired if attention down
	Insight	May be preserved

EXAMINATION
General appearance
Look for general medical illness

INVESTIGATIONS
Exclude organic disease
FBC / ESR / U&E / Calcium / TFT
ECG if palpitations

TREATMENT
If suicidal may need to 'section' under Mental Health Act

Drugs   Re-uptake inhibitors
                 Tricyclics   Imipramine / Clomipramine
                                 Prothiaden / Lofepramine /
                                 Amitriptyline
                 Serotonin   Fluoxetine / Paroxetine / Citalopram /
                                 Sertraline
                 Monoamine oxidase inhibitors (second line)
                                 Phenelzine (old)
                                 Moclobemide (new)

Electroconvulsive treatment if psychotic depression
Psychological treatment (cognitive therapy)

Comment
Often patients with anxiety neurosis develop depression and
features of both conditions co-exist. During the history you must
look for symptoms for anxiety, eg:

Palpitations	Tachycardia	Bowel disturbance	Sweating
Irritability	Muscle pain	Swallowing problems	Phobias
Panic attacks	Agoraphobia	Pins and needles	Dizziness

Be sure to elucidate any thyroid or cardiac disease and check
whether the patient is using β-agonist inhalers.
Phaeochromocytoma is very rare. Treatment involves anxiety
management and anti-depressant drugs.

Case 102:
PSYCHOSIS / SCHIZOPHRENIA

PC   'What has been going on in your life recently?'

HPC   Prodromal phase   Loss of interest / Poor hygiene / Change in mood / Decline in function

The interview should find out whether there are any of the diagnostic features of schizophrenia (see Teaching points) and also exclude mania, depression, intoxication and organic brain syndromes including epilepsy.

Look for precipitating factors / Recent life events

PMH   Previous episodes of psychiatric disease
Deafness / blindness (in elderly)

FH   Positive family history is common

Personal   Birth trauma
Erratic performance at school, especially boys
Unable to have long-term relationship
Poor employment record
Criminal record
Low income etc.
Poor housing / living rough

Premorbid   Schizoid / Schizotypal personality / Withdrawn / Eccentric / Paranoid

Drugs   Treatment ? depot injections
Cannabis / Amphetamines precipitate psychotic illness
Prescribed medication, eg iv steroids

Smoking

Alcohol   May be excessive

ROS   ? Epilepsy / Headaches (brain tumour) / Alcohol
            withdrawal

Mental state Behaviour   Self-neglect / Abnormal movements
                             (treatment effects)
                Speech   Varied / Incomprehensible /
                             Neologisms
                Mood   Blunted affect / Inappropriate affect
                             (excess laughing etc.)
                Thought   Insertion / Withdrawal /
                             Broadcasting / Abnormal beliefs
                             (belief that they are Jesus Christ) / In
                             contact with TV set
                Perception   Auditory hallucinations third person
                             / Thought echo / Running
                             commentary / Passivity feelings
                Orientation ? Jesus Christ / In contact with TV set
                             / Often normal
                Attention   Often poor
                Memory   Decreased if concentration poor
                Insight   Depends on degree of treatment

NB: Some forms of schizophrenia have more negative features –
poverty of speech / Slow thought, etc.

EXAMINATION
General appearance
            Signs of drug use / Brain tumour

INVESTIGATIONS
            Psychosocial investigations
            Drug screen / EEG / CT scan
TREATMENT
            Drugs   Acute   Neuroleptic drugs, eg
                                  chlorpromazine
                       Chronic   Oral / Depot, eg flupentixol
            Supportive Decreased stress in the environment
                       Decreased expressed emotion in family
            Rehabilitation
                       Day care

Comment

The diagnosis of schizophrenia is indicated by one or more of the following symptoms:

Disorders of: Thought possession
             Thought insertion
             Thought withdrawal
             Thought broadcasting
Auditory hallucinations in which the person hears:
             His own thoughts out loud (thought echo)
             People discussing him in the third person
             Voices forming a running commentary
Passivity feelings
             Feeling under control of an outside influence
Delusions
             Persistent delusions culturally / Physically impossible
             Delusional perception
Or two or more of the following:
             Persistent hallucinations
             Incoherent / Irrelevant speech / Mannerisms /
             Neologisms
             Catatonic phenomena
             Negative symptoms

For further details of Psychosis/schizophrenia and other psychiatric diseases we suggest referring to Goldberg D, Benjamin S, Creed F. Psychiatry in Medical Practice, Taylor and Francis Ltd 1994.

Case 103:
ANOREXIA NERVOSA

PC   When was the condition first brought to medical attention? Why?

HPC   Fat in past
How has patient dieted or controlled calories
Ask about exercise (usually excessive)
Previous investigations for diarrhoea / Metabolic problems / Amenorrhoea
Ask about body image / Fear of fatness
Bulimic episodes
Menstrual history

PMH   Diabetes / Thyroid disease

FH   Increased eating disorders in family members

Personal   Disturbed family relationships
Avoidance of maturity including sexual relationships
Denial of family problems
Parental discord (divorce / separation)

Drugs   Laxatives / Diuretics

Smoking

Alcohol

ROS   Raynaud's phenomenon is common
Excess hair (lanugo) on face and back
Feel cold
Exclude differential conditions:
Diabetes
Weight loss – hyperthyroidism / Inflammatory bowel disease
Amenorrhoea – Ovarian / Pituitary disease

Mental state	Behaviour	Normal
	Speech	Normal
	Mood	Anxious / Depressed / Unconcerned about health
	Thought	Abnormal body image / May be suicidal
	Perception	
	Orientation	
	Attention	
	Memory	
	Insight	Lacking regarding health

EXAMINATION
General appearance

Thin / Cold peripheries / Lanugo hair
Ask for weight and height and calculate body mass dex (weight in kg divided by height in m^2)
Note the absence of hyperthyroidism etc.

INVESTIGATIONS

Social investigation of family relationships
Glucose / Thyroid function tests
U&E (low K$^+$ with purgatives or diuretics)
Low serum protein / Follicle-stimulating hormone, luteinising hormone decreased / ACTH increased (stress response)

TREATMENT

Restore body weight
Behavioural programme, progressive introduction of rewards for weight gain
Psychotherapy   Family therapy for younger patients
Individual therapy if older
May need to move away from family situation (inpatient / other carer)
May need anti-depressant medication

Case 104:
SUBSTANCE ABUSE

This may relate to any drug but more often than not it applies to alcohol in which case there is an overlap with chronic liver disease. There develops a **compulsion** to use the drug, **increased tolerance** and **withdrawal symptoms** on stopping. You must look out for physical, psychological and social complications, eg chronic liver disease, changes in mood, convictions and marriage breakdown and salience or stereotyped behaviour.

PC	When first brought to medical attention? Why?

HPC	When first took the drug and when became used regularly or more heavily (? amount)
	Why did they first use the drug?
	    Peer pressure / Anxiety / Depression / Availability
	What effects did and does the drug have?
	When first had problems with the drug / What problems?
	    How do they obtain (and pay for) the drug / How do they use it (inject / Smoke etc)?
	How has tolerance developed?
	What withdrawal effects are noticed? Fits / Delirium tremens / Cold turkey / Anxiety
	What other symptoms of dependence?

PMH	Depression or other psychiatric history Chronic illness or chronic pain
FH	Increased addictive behaviour in family members
Personal	Childhood exposure to addictive behaviour / Abuse / Neglected childhood Poor performance at school if glue sniffer Poor employment record / **High risk occupation** (Barman / Traveller / Medic) Criminal record Theft / Violence / Drink Driving / Prostitution Poor marital history (Divorce / Aggression) Poor standard of living as money goes on drug habit

Premorbid

Drugs   Any medication

Smoking   Signs of addictive behaviour

Alcohol

Number of units per week / Typical drinking day
The CAGE questionnaire indicates excessive drinking
if there are two or more yes answers.

C   Have you ever felt you ought to **C**ut down on
your drinking?

A   Have people **A**nnoyed you by criticising your
drinking?

G   Have you ever felt **G**uilty about your drinking?

E   Have you ever had a drink first thing in the
morning to steady your nerves or get rid of a
hangover (**E**ye opener)?

ROS   Here you must identify any associations with the
particular drug. Chronic liver disease with alcohol
and AIDS with iv drug use etc.
Chest infections / Cardiomyopathy / Endocarditis
with iv drug abuse
Gastritis / Oesophagitis / Pancreatitis / Hepatitis
Stroke / Neuropathy / Cerebellar degeneration /
Myopathy / Head injury / Korsakoff's / Wernicke's
syndromes with alcohol

Mental state

Behaviour	Poor self-care / Abnormal movements / Withdrawal symptoms
Speech	Cerebellar / Slurred
Mood	Anxiety / Depression
Thought	Suicide / Preoccupation with drugs / Paranoid ideas
Perception	
Orientation	Abnormal if intoxicated (hopefully not during exam)
Attention	Poor

Memory	Korsakoff's – poor retrograde memory
Insight	'I can kick it'; but they can't

EXAMINATION
General appearance
Signs of the complications of the substance used
Needle marks / Phlebitis
AIDS
Chronic liver disease

INVESTIGATIONS
FBC, U&E, LFT and others depending on type of drug
Social investigations

TREATMENT

Acute	Treatment of withdrawal	
	Alcohol	Chlordiazepoxide regimen
	Opiates	Symptomatic / Methadone
Long term	Psychological support / Alcoholics Anonymous Antabuse Methadone	

Other treatment of underlying mood disorder

Comments
The drugs most often abused are: Alcohol / Opiates / Hallucinogens / Amphetamines / Cannabis / Solvents. There may be a history of abuse of several drugs over the course of the illness and each of these should be mentioned.

OTHER COMMON PSYCHIATRIC LONG CASES
As part of your revision you may wish to make up similar long case plans for the other common cases:

* Mania / Anxiety / Obsessive compulsive disorders / Personality disorder / Dementia / Korsakoff's syndrome

HIV / AIDS

105   HIV Infection / Aids

Case 105:
HIV INFECTION / AIDS

Since the first edition of this book human immunodeficiency virus (HIV) infection/Acquired immune deficiency syndrome (AIDS) has become, unfortunately, much more common. We have therefore included some notes on the common features that we feel you should know about.

A chronic retroviral infection with complications affecting every organ system.

The patient may tell you they are HIV positive, and may be highly informed about their clinical history, viral load and treatment.

Alternatively they may present with a history and signs of a condition suggesting underlying HIV infection, and there may be identifiable risk factors for HIV exposure.

Seroconversion illness

Occurs in 25–65%
A non-specific transient glandular fever-like illness at the time of antibody formation, within three months of viral inoculation. Other features may include rash, meningitis, Guillain–Barré syndrome or even encephalitis.

Common manifestations of advanced HIV infection/AIDS

Careful general examination including skin, eyes and mouth may reveal a number of the features below, and there may be a history of one or more of the specific organ system infections/ malignancies.

General – weight loss, anorexia, muscle wasting, generalised lymphadenopathy, non-Hodgkin's lymphoma from variety of sites

Skin – seborrhoeic dermatitis, recurrent shingles (often different dermatomes), molluscum contagiosum, Kaposi's sarcoma, intractable viral warts, recurrent staphylococcal infection

Mouth – oral hairy leukoplakia, oropharyngeal candidiasis, recurrent ulceration, widespread herpes simplex infection

Respiratory – recurrent bacterial pneumonia, Pneumocystis carinii pneumonia (PCP), tuberculosis, fungal pneumonia

Gastrointestinal – oesophageal candidiasis, cryptosporidiosis (diarrhoea), sclerosing cholangitis

Anogenital – invasive cervical carcinoma, herpes simplex, anogenital warts, symptoms of concurrent sexually transmitted diseases (STDs)

Neurological – cerebral toxoplasmosis, cryptococcal meningitis, progressive multifocal leucoencephalopathy (PML) due to JC virus, peripheral neuropathy, HIV-dementia complex, CNS lymphoma

Ocular – cytomegalovirus (CMV) retinitis

Modes of viral transmission

- Male homosexual transmission (commonest route in UK)
- Intravenous drug needle sharing/Needlestick injuries
- Contaminated blood products/Donor organs
- Mother to child transmission
- Heterosexual transmission (commonest route in Africa, increasing in UK)

Treatment

- Specific treatments for individual opportunistic infections/Malignancies
- Highly active anti-retroviral treatment (HAART) has markedly improved life expectancy
- Treatment effectiveness judged by HIV viral load measurement
- Worldwide, majority of those infected have no access to treatment: socio-political ramifications.

MISCELLANEOUS VIVA QUESTIONS

Tell me about the genetics of myotonic dystrophy.

Myotonic dystrophy is an autosomal dominant disorder characterised by myotonia, muscle dystrophy, hypogonadism, frontal balding and cardiac involvement. The genetic mutation in myotonic dystrophy is an expanded trinucleotide repeat on chromosome 19. The severity of the condition varies with the number of repeats: normal individuals carry 5–30 repeat copies, mildly affected patients from 50–80 and severely affected individuals 2000 or more copies. Like some other autosomal dominant disorders it shows variable penetrance. Similarly it shows anticipation – an increase in severity of disease in successive generations. Patients with affected mothers are more severely affected than those with affected fathers, and the rare severe congenital form of the disease almost exclusively occurs in offspring of affected mothers.(Case 65)

What do you understand by the term autosomal recessive?

Autosomal recessive disorders occur in a person whose healthy parents both carry the same recessive gene. The risk of recurrence for future pregnancies is 25% (1 in 4). Unlike autosomal dominant disorders there is usually no family history of the disease.

Consanguinity increases the risk of a recessive disorder because both parents are more likely to carry the same defective gene, which has been inherited from a common ancestor.

Cystic fibrosis is the commonest autosomal recessive disease in the UK, with a carrier frequency of 1 in 20.

Many of the inborn errors of metabolism are autosomal recessive disorders.

Tell me about the genetics of cystic fibrosis

Cystic fibrosis is the commonest autosomal recessive disorder in northern Europeans; 1 in 20 of the population is a carrier, giving a disease frequency of approximately 1 in 2000 live born infants. Hundreds of different mutations in the cystic fibrosis gene (on chromosome 7) have been found, but one common mutation accounts for over 70% of all cases.

When both partners are carriers there is a 1 in 4 risk to each pregnancy of having a child with cystic fibrosis. Precise prenatal diagnosis is possible, and selective termination of affected pregnancies can be offered, if desired.

How would you break the news to someone that they had motor neurone disease?

Very importantly this should take place in a quiet environment, preferably not during a busy round on a noisy ward. The news should be imparted by the most senior member of the medical team, the consultant, and the nurse looking after the patient/MND nurse specialist should ideally be present. It is probably best to give the patient advance notice that you are going to talk to them about the results of their investigations, and encourage them to invite a family member to be there.

Most patients will probably not be familiar with motor neurone disease. It should be explained that it is a progressive condition affecting the nerves that supply the muscles, leading to the wasting and weakness, which presumably they have presented with. They should be told that there is a treatment available (riluzole) which may slow the rate of progression of the disease, but that it is not a curative treatment. Explain that the cause remains unknown, although there is a great deal of research in progress. Explain that in the vast majority of cases it is not familial.

Offer the patient, and family, literature/Patient leaflets on the condition, but do not foist these upon them.

It is important to arrange a follow-up appointment in the near future, as undoubtedly they will have a lot of questions when they have had time to reflect upon the diagnosis and its implications.

What advice would you give to a patient going on a long flight to Australia?

Assuming the patient is otherwise well, he can be reassured that the risks of developing a DVT are low, and can be minimised by taking the following steps:

regular movement of the feet and legs while sitting
taking frequent walks around the cabin
liberal consumption on non-alcoholic beverages
wearing of well fitting compression stockings.
The routine use of aspirin is not recommended, because of the
high incidence of gastrointestinal side-effects.
High-risk patients may need low-molecular weight heparin, and
specialist advice should be sought.

What would you look for in a blood count to tell you the cause of anaemia?

One would look for platelet and white counts to make sure that one is not dealing with pancytopenia, myelo/lymphoproliferative disorder, eg high white count, low platelets of chronic lymphoid leukemia in an elderly patient or pancytopenia in an elderly patient suggesting myelodysplasia. If these are normal one can look at the red cell MCV to see if microcytic, normocytic or macrocytic, eg iron deficiency, anaemia of chronic disease and B_{12} deficiency, respectively. If MCV is too low for level of anaemia suspect thalassaemia.

Give me some causes of raised sodium. Give me some causes of lowered sodium.

Hypernatraemia is most commonly due to predominant water loss from inadequate fluid replacement, insensible loss due to febrile illness, diarrhoea or urinary loss due to diuretic, osmotic diuresis in diabetes or hypercalcaemia.

Hyponatraemia is best considered in the context of the patient's extra-cellular fluid volume:
   Hypovolaemic causes include burns, D+V, pancreatitis, Addison's disease, salt wasting nephropathy, cerebral salt wasting
   Euvolaemic: Spurious due to high plasma protein or triglycerides, sickle cell, hyperglycaemia, SIADH, ACTH deficiency
   Hypervolaemic(oedematous):Cirrhosis, cardiac failure, nephrotic syndrome, renal failure.

Discuss screening.

Screening usually involves testing large numbers of apparently healthy people to find those who have a specified disease or condition and those who do not. The sensitivity and specificity of the test will determine the success. It is usually only thought to be ethical to screen if there is appropriate treatment available, eg cervical smears, mammography, Guthrie test.

What is the placebo response?

This is a positive therapeutic response by a patient when treated by an inactive or ineffective therapy (physical, medical, psychological or surgical).

How would you use a placebo response in a clinical trial?

The clinical response to placebo treatment is compared to the clinical response to active treatment usually with the patient and the doctor ignorant as to which preparation the patient is taking (double-blind). Only if there is a statistically significant benefit of the active treatment over the placebo will the treatment be declared beneficial.

What do you mean by a normal population?

This assumes for any measurement that the population is distributed in a Gaussian distribution – 95% within ± 2 standard deviations of the mean.

What do confidence intervals represent?

Confidence intervals represent the level that is set to say whether statistically an event is more or less likely to happen by chance than after a certain treatment, ie 95% confidence interval means that there is only a 5% (1 in 20 chance) that a result occurred by chance and a 19/20 chance that the result is real.

What would you do when called to a patient who was unconscious?

Resuscitation is the first step: protection of the airway, respiration, and circulatory support (ABC case 00). You will need help. Send blood for glucose, biochemistry and toxicology, and then administer iv glucose.

Obtain as much history as possible from family/friends. Did the patient suddenly collapse, had they been unwell for the preceding few days, are thy known to take alcohol/drugs?

Examination is directed to finding the cause as well as assessing the level of unconsciousness (using the Glasgow Coma Scale). Look for fever, neck stiffness and rash suggestive of meningitis, any bruising to suggest trauma, widely dilated pupils secondary to drug intoxication?

The presence of focal neurological signs suggests an intracranial structural cause, eg haematoma, and the patient will require urgent CT scanning.

How would you manage a young girl with an acute asthma attack?

First assess the severity of the asthma attack. Features indicative of a severe attack are: respiratory rate > 25, tachycardia > 110, inability to complete full sentences and peak expiratory flow (PEF) < 50% best/predicted.

Then treatment should be given with high-flow oxygen, nebulised bronchodilators and steroids. If the attack is severe the patient should be admitted.

Ask the patient about their compliance with their treatment, especially inhaled steroids, and stress the importance of regular treatment.

You are called to an unconscious patient. On investigation you find they have ventricular fibrillation; outline your initial management.

See Case 14
Confirm patient unconscious and ensure help is on the way.
Remember ABC – airway, breathing, circulation.

Ensure adequate airway and oxygenation, preferably via an endotracheal tube.

Ensure defibrillator electrodes applied correctly, ask others to stand clear and deliver first shock (200 J). If ventricular fibrillation* persists deliver further shocks (200 J, then 360 J).

Continue cardiac massage for 1 minute.

Re-check rhythm and repeat cycle of defibrillation and cardiac massage.

Administer adrenaline (1:10 000 × 10 ml) every 3 minutes via large vein, adequately flushed by normal saline.

Correct reversible causes, eg hypo/hyperkalaemia.

*Ventricular fibrillation is the commonest primary arrhythmia at the start of cardiac arrest. Survival is crucially dependent on minimising the delay before delivering a countershock.

Tell me about some emergencies you have seen in the Accident and Emergency Department

This is up to you start with something you know about eg myocardial infarction.

INDEX